Ronald E. Hellman, MD
Jack Drescher, MD
Editors

Handbook of LGBT Issues in Community Mental Health

Handbook of LGBT Issues in Community Mental Health has been co-published simultaneously as *Journal of Gay & Lesbian Psychotherapy*, Volume 8, Numbers 3/4 2004.

Pre-publication REVIEWS, COMMENTARIES, EVALUATIONS . . .

"COMPREHENSIVE . . . Essential reading for all mental health professionals, gay or straight. . . . Written by leaders in the field. . . . RICHLY STREWN WITH DATA, USEFUL ADDRESSES OF VOLUNTARY AND OTHER ORGANIZATIONS, AND CASE HISTORIES. . . . Documents the efforts of ordinary LBG people to organize public funding for the services they needed, how services have developed for LGB people with serious and enduring mental illness, the mental health problems suffered by some LGB adolescents, and the complex issues that face transgendered people."

Michael King, MD, PhD, FRCP, FRCGP, FRCPsych
Professor of Primary Care Psychiatry
Department of Mental Health Sciences
Royal Free and University
College Medical School, London

Handbook
of LGBT Issues
in Community
Mental Health

Handbook of LGBT Issues in Community Mental Health has been co-published simultaneously as *Journal of Gay & Lesbian Psychotherapy*, Volume 8, Numbers 3/4 2004.

The *Journal of Gay & Lesbian Psychotherapy* Monographic "Separates"

Below is a list of "separates," which in serials librarianship means a special issue simultaneously published as a special journal issue or double-issue *and* as a "separate" hardbound monograph. (This is a format which we also call a "DocuSerial.")

"Separates" are published because specialized libraries or professionals may wish to purchase a specific thematic issue by itself in a format which can be separately cataloged and shelved, as opposed to purchasing the journal on an on-going basis. Faculty members may also more easily consider a "separate" for classroom adoption.

"Separates" are carefully classified separately with the major book jobbers so that the journal tie-in can be noted on new book order slips to avoid duplicate purchasing.

You may wish to visit Haworth's website at . . .

http://www.HaworthPress.com

. . . to search our online catalog for complete tables of contents of these separates and related publications.

You may also call 1-800-HAWORTH (outside US/Canada: 607-722-5857), or Fax: 1-800-895-0582 (outside US/Canada: 607-771-0012), or e-mail at:

docdelivery@haworthpress.com

Handbook of LGBT Issues in Community Mental Health, edited by Ronald E. Hellman, MD, and Jack Drescher, MD (Vol. 8, No. 3/4, 2004). *"COMPREHENSIVE . . . Richly strewn with data, useful addresses of voluntary and other organizations, and case histories." (Michael King, MD, PhD, Professor of Primary Care Psychiatry, Royal Free and University College Medical School, London)*

Transgender Subjectivities: A Clinician's Guide, edited by Ubaldo Leli, MD, and Jack Drescher, MD (Vol. 8, No. 1/2, 2004). *"INDISPENSABLE for diagnosticians and therapists dealing with gender dysphoria, important for researchers, and a direct source of help for all individuals suffering from painful uncertainties regarding their sexual identity." (Otto F. Kernberg, MD, Director, Personality Disorders Institute, Weill Medical College of Cornell University)*

The Mental Health Professions and Homosexuality: International Perspectives, edited by Vittorio Lingiardi, MD, and Jack Drescher, MD (Vol. 7, No. 1/2, 2003). *"PROVIDES A WORLDWIDE PERSPECTIVE that illuminates the psychiatric, psychoanalytic, and mental health professions' understanding and treatment of both lay and professional sexual minorities." (Bob Barrett, PhD, Professor and Counseling Program Coordinator, University of North Carolina at Charlotte)*

Sexual Conversion Therapy: Ethical, Clinical, and Research Perspectives, edited by Ariel Shidlo, PhD, Michael Schroeder, PsyD, and Jack Drescher, MD (Vol. 5, No. 3/4, 2001). *"THIS IS AN IMPORTANT BOOK. . . . AN INVALUABLE RESOURCES FOR MENTAL HEALTH PROVIDERS AND POLICYMAKERS. This book gives voice to those men and women who have experienced painful, degrading, and unsuccessful conversion therapy and survived. The ethics and misuses of conversion therapy practice are well documented, as are the harmful effects." (Joyce Hunter, DSW, Research Scientist, HIV Center for Clinical & Behavioral Studies, New York State Psychiatric Institute/Columbia University, New York City)*

Gay and Lesbian Parenting, edited by Deborah F. Glazer, PhD, and Jack Drescher, MD (Vol. 4, No. 3/4, 2001). *Richly textured, probing. These papers accomplish a rare feat: they explore in a candid, psychologically sophisticated, yet highly readable fashion how parenthood impacts lesbian and gay identity and how these identities affect the experience of parenting. Wonderfully informative. (Martin Stephen Frommer, PhD, Faculty/Supervisor, The Institute for Contemporary Psychotherapy, New York City).*

Addictions in the Gay and Lesbian Community, edited by Jeffrey R. Guss, MD, and Jack Drescher, MD (Vol. 3, No. 3/4, 2000). *Explores the unique clinical considerations involved in addiction treatment for gay men and lesbians, groups that reportedly use and abuse alcohol and substances at higher rates than the general population.*

Handbook of LGBT Issues in Community Mental Health

Ronald E. Hellman, MD
Jack Drescher, MD
Editors

Handbook of LGBT Issues in Community Mental Health has been
co-published simultaneously as *Journal of Gay & Lesbian
Psychotherapy*, Volume 8, Numbers 3/4 2004.

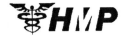

The Haworth Medical Press®
Harrington Park Press®
Imprints of The Haworth Press, Inc.

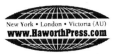

New York • London • Victoria (AU)
www.HaworthPress.com

Published by

The Haworth Medical Press®, 10 Alice Street, Binghamton, NY 13904-1580 USA

The Haworth Medical Press® is an imprint of The Haworth Press, Inc., 10 Alice Street, Binghamton, NY 13904-1580 USA.

Handbook of LGBT Issues in Community Mental Health has been co-published simultaneously as *Journal of Gay & Lesbian Psychotherapy*, Volume 8, Numbers 3/4 2004.

The development, preparation, and publication of this work has been undertaken with great care. However, the publisher, employees, editors, and agents of The Haworth Press and all imprints of The Haworth Press, Inc., including The Haworth Medical Press® and Pharmaceutical Products Press®, are not responsible for any errors contained herein or for consequences that may ensue from use of materials or information contained in this work. Opinions expressed by the author(s) are not necessarily those of The Haworth Press, Inc. With regard to case studies, identities and circumstances of individuals discussed herein have been changed to protect confidentiality. Any resemblance to actual persons, living or dead, is entirely coincidental.

Cover design by Marylouise E. Doyle

Library of Congress Cataloging-in-Publication Data

Handbook of LGBT issues in community mental health / Ronald E. Hellman, Jack Drescher, editors.
       p. ; cm.
       Co-published simultaneously as Journal of gay & lesbian psychotherapy, Volume 8, Numbers 3/4, 2004.
       Includes bibliographical references and index.
       ISBN 0-7890-2309-1 (hard cover : alk. paper) – ISBN 0-7890-2310-5 (soft cover : alk. paper)
       1. Community mental health services. 2. Gays–Mental health. 3. Bisexuals–Mental health. 4. Transsexuals–Mental health. 5. Community psychiatry.
       [DNLM: 1. Community Mental Health Services. 2. Homosexuality. 3. Bisexuality. 4. Community Psychiatry–methods. 5. Cultural Diversity. 6. Transsexualism.] I. Title: Handbook of lesbian, gay, bisexual, transgender issues in community mental health. II. Hellman, Ronald E. III. Drescher, Jack, 1951- IV. Journal of gay & lesbian psychotherapy
RC451.4.G39H36 2004
362.2'2'08664–dc22
                                                                                    2004016722

Indexing, Abstracting & Website/Internet Coverage

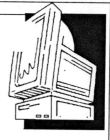

This section provides you with a list of major indexing & abstracting services and other tools for bibliographic access. That is to say, each service began covering this periodical during the year noted in the right column. Most Websites which are listed below have indicated that they will either post, disseminate, compile, archive, cite or alert their own Website users with research-based content from this work. (This list is as current as the copyright date of this publication.)

Abstracting, Website/Indexing Coverage . . . . Year When Coverage Began

- *Abstracts in Anthropology* 1991
- *Academic Index (on-line)* 1992
- *Academic Search Elite (EBSCO)* 1998
- *Academic Search Premier (EBSCO)* 2001
- *Business Source Corporate: coverage of nearly 3,350 quality magazines and journals; designed to meet the diverse information needs of corporations; EBSCO Publishing <http://www.epnet.com/corporate/bsourcecorp.asp>* 1998
- *Contemporary Women's Issues* 1998
- *e-psyche, LLC <http://www.e-psyche.net>* 2001
- *Expanded Academic ASAP <http://www.galegroup.com>* 1993
- *Expanded Academic ASAP–International <http://www.galegroup.com>* 1993
- *Expanded Academic Index* 1995
- *Family Index Database <http://www.familyscholar.com>* 2003
- *Family Violence & Sexual Assault Bulletin* 1992
- *GenderWatch <http://www.slinfo.com>* 1999
- *GLBT Life, EBSCO Publishing <http://www.epnet.com/academic/glbt.asp>* 2004

(continued)

   *Exact start date to come.

Special Bibliographic Notes related to special journal issues
(separates) and indexing/abstracting:

- indexing/abstracting services in this list will also cover material in any "separate" that is co-published simultaneously with Haworth's special thematic journal issue or DocuSerial. Indexing/abstracting usually covers material at the article/chapter level.
- monographic co-editions are intended for either non-subscribers or libraries which intend to purchase a second copy for their circulating collections.
- monographic co-editions are reported to all jobbers/wholesalers/approval plans. The source journal is listed as the "series" to assist the prevention of duplicate purchasing in the same manner utilized for books-in-series.
- to facilitate user/access services all indexing/abstracting services are encouraged to utilize the co-indexing entry note indicated at the bottom of the first page of each article/chapter/contribution.
- this is intended to assist a library user of any reference tool (whether print, electronic, online, or CD-ROM) to locate the monographic version if the library has purchased this version but not a subscription to the source journal.
- individual articles/chapters in any Haworth publication are also available through the Haworth Document Delivery Service (HDDS).

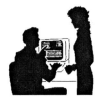

Handbook of LGBT Issues in Community Mental Health

CONTENTS

ABOUT THE EDITORS

Ronald Hellman, MD, is Director of the LGBT Affirmative Program at South Beach Psychiatric Center in Brooklyn, New York.

Jack Drescher, MD, is a Fellow, Training and Supervising Analyst at the William Alanson White Psychoanalytic Institute. He is Past President of the New York County District Branch, American Psychiatric Association and Chair of the Committee on GLB Concerns of the APA. Author of *Psychoanalytic Therapy and the Gay Man* (1998, The Analytic Press), and Editor-in-Chief of the *JGLP*, Dr. Drescher is in private practice in New York City.

Coming Out in the Public Sector:
Introduction

While it was once estimated that gay people represented ten percent of the adult US population (Kinsey, Pomeroy and Martin, 1948; Kinsey et al., 1953), more reliable and recent data estimates the prevalence of homosexuality between 1 and 5% (Laumann et al., 1994).[1] Although it would be natural to assume that some portion of a population of untold millions would find its way into the public mental health sector, one would be hard pressed to make a case for the mental health needs of these individuals–or even of their very existence–based on the existing public health literature.

This invisibility of gay people in the mental health public sector is disturbing, but not altogether surprising. In fact, the treatment of lesbian, gay, bisexual and transgender (LGBT) individuals in public psychiatric institutions reflects a long history of changing cultural views and values which have influenced core concepts of mental illness and sexuality. Public psychiatric institutions are products of governmental bodies, and their history illuminates the role of government in relation to mental illness and sexuality.

Until the mid-1800s, individuals with serious mental illness languished in poorhouses and prisons. Although sympathetic care of the mentally ill had existed during the classical era in Greece, and was recorded through significant periods of Western civilization (Alexander and Selesnick, 1966), it did not generally exist in the early days of the United States. State-funded asylums were later established in the mid-1800s to redress this situation due to the reform efforts of Dorothea Dix and others (Mora, 1975). Over the next century, however, these public institutions received little financial support, and they developed a reputation for neglect and overcrowding.

[Haworth co-indexing entry note]: "Coming Out in the Public Sector: Introduction." Hellman, Ronald E., and Jack Drescher. Co-published simultaneously in *Journal of Gay & Lesbian Psychotherapy* (The Haworth Medical Press, an imprint of The Haworth Press, Inc.) Vol. 8, No. 3/4, 2004, pp. 1-9; and: *Handbook of LGBT Issues in Community Mental Health* (ed: Ronald E. Hellman, and Jack Drescher) The Haworth Medical Press, an imprint of The Haworth Press, Inc., 2004, pp. 1-9. Single or multiple copies of this article are available for a fee from The Haworth Document Delivery Service [1-800-HAWORTH, 9:00 a.m. - 5:00 p.m. (EST). E-mail address: docdelivery@haworthpress.com].

http://www.haworthpress.com/web/JGLP
Digital Object Identifier: 10.1300/J236v08n03_01

1

Exposure of the inhumane conditions in state institutions resulted in political pressure that inevitably moved the federal government to become involved in the improvement of care for the mentally ill. Congress passed the Public Health Service Act of 1944, which committed the federal government to provide state grants and research funding to advance mental health service provision. In 1963, Congress established the Community Mental Health Centers Act, which authorized a new form of public sector mental health care delivery through local community based centers–a system that continues today. Federal funding of mental health treatment through Medicare and Medicaid followed in 1965 (Kent and Gibson, 1992).

Separate public and private health care systems evolved in the mid-twentieth century with the widespread development of private health insurance plans. As a result, some agencies grew into mixed systems with both government and non-governmental revenue sources. Individuals lacking insurance, who required care beyond insurance coverage limits, or who were unable to pay "out of pocket" could receive treatment through public state psychiatric hospitals, local general hospitals, and community mental health centers. Veterans of the armed forces could also receive care through the Veteran's Administration (VA) hospitals and clinics. Disabled individuals with little to no income could receive coverage under federal Supplemental Security Income (SSI), while those with a work history under Social Security would receive Social Security Disability (SSD) coverage.

More recently, economic pressure has resulted in hybrid programs to manage mental health care. In some public programs, state agencies purchase care from private organizations rather than provide it directly. These behavioral health care programs are managed separately, or "carved out" to these private organizations. Although such plans may contain costs, there is preliminary evidence that they are associated with disruptions in the continuity of care, lower levels of medication compliance, and inadequate provision of ancillary services (Mechanic, 2003). Thus, future modification in the structure and administration of the public mental health sector is a virtual certainty.

Because governments are the major source of funding and administration of treatment programs for those with serious mental illness, these public agencies are able to exert a sizable influence over the parameters of treatment through regulations, guidelines, licensing, and accreditation. Those in politically powerful positions can also transmit their ethical values, and thereby influence treatment, through the choices they make when they cast their ballot on particular governmental budget allocations, grants, discretionary funds, and related legislation. The political process is, therefore, an intimate component of the development and support of public sector mental health programs. By contrast, private agencies are responsible to a board of directors or trustees, may be investor-owned, and respond to the market place in order to provide services that will generate a profit (Talbott and Hales, 2002).

Because of the differences in the way they function, public and private systems have the potential to complement each other in addressing a broad range of mental health care needs from within the LGBT population. How effectively they do this is yet to be determined. Public and private agencies can serve diverse groups and socioeconomic strata in the LGBT community, depending on their philosophy and revenue sources, but the quality of LGBT specific care largely remains a self-regulated affair.

Irrespective of the sector that is served, developing LGBT focused mental health programs is challenging. Differences in leadership and administrative structures, financial risk, developmental phase of the enterprise, philosophy, and targeted subcultures result in organizations with distinct characteristics and varying longevity. Thus, there is no single model for program structure, although all must function in ways that incorporate accepted standards of mental health treatment and culturally relevant service practices.

The actual role of the public psychiatric system in the provision of mental health services to LGBT individuals remains to be determined. The historical background is quite complex because, as we see today, the subject is at the interface between a range of issues, including religious belief, government, science, civil rights, sexuality and mental health.

Historically, the nascent role of government in the American colonies was strongly influenced by the religious background of early European settlers. Pre-colonial settlers, observing "sodomy" among Native Americans, cited the need for eradication of these behaviors as a justification for colonization (Katz, 1983). With further establishment of the East coast territories, public standards of morality were enforced by the new governments and included the regulation of sexual and gender behavior (Altman, 1982).

During those early days of European settlement, there were no categories of "homosexual" or "mentally ill" persons as they are understood today. Family and community were organizing sources of personal identity in a world where procreation and survival were paramount. No distinction existed between emotions, behavior, and sexual orientation. Feelings were considered inner acts of the soul. Sodomy was categorized as a subset of lust that included any human desire that opposed God's work. The soul could be possessed by the devil, leading to symptoms recognized today as mental illness (Katz, 1983).

With the coming of the Enlightenment of the eighteenth century, observation and reason, rather than faith, magical thinking, and tradition gained prominence in efforts to understand mental illness and sexuality. Some have argued that sexual discourse became the powerful, new tool of the medical establishment (Foucault, 1978). Over the next two centuries, sexual differences were scrutinized through the lens of scientific inquiry and subjected to categorization, analysis, and remediation. Homosexuality was treated as an illness, both in private settings and public institutions. Those who "suffered" from it were either consigned to the psychoanalyst's offices with their old world charm (Bieber et al., 1962), or engaged as a subject of clinical research in major academic centers supported by government grants (Weinberg and Bell, 1972). Virtually all clinical textbooks before 1970 viewed homosexuality as a pathological entity (Silverstein, 1995).

A combination of scientific inquiry and political activism changed all that. Homosexuality was "liberated" from the chains of pathological discourse when the American Psychiatric Association removed it from its diagnostic manual, the *DSM*, in 1973 (Bayer, 1981; Hire, 2002; Scasta, 2002; Drescher, 2003; Rosario, 2003; Sbordone, 2003). For the mental health mainstream, a paradigm shift (Kuhn, 1972) had occurred rather suddenly. However, translating this theoretical shift into practical applications in the public sector has taken much longer. Johnsgard and Schumacher (1970) were probably the first authors to describe an affirmative treatment approach for those with homosexual concerns. The first affirmative treatment methods that were applied to LGBT individuals in a public psychiatric institution appear to have occurred in the early 1970s at Atascadaro State Hospital in California. There, an openly gay subculture was allowed to thrive. Gay students from the community were brought in to role model gay social skills. A gay consciousness-raising group was formed which met on a regular basis and same-sex dancing was allowed at ward parties (Thompson, 1994).

Definitions of sanity are inextricably linked to social and cultural norms (Grob, 1994). These norms guide the valuation of scientific data, which, in turn, influence social ethical standards. Despite the 1973 change in APA outlook, and the sporadic endeavor in public psychiatric settings, there has been a lack of any broad, organized effort to deliver gay affirmative mental health care in the public sector. This may be a function of either neglect, bias (Group for the Advancement of Psychiatry, 2000), or both.

Contemporary support of affirmative LGBT mental health programs by governments, although still uncommon, represents a novel turn in the annals of civic life. The primary stimulus for change has come at the state governmental level where the impetus to provide culturally competent mental health treatment to culturally diverse groups now includes sexual minorities (McCarn, 1999; NASMHPD, 2000). However, as yet, there is no uniformly mandated governmental response to the mental health concerns of sexual minorities.

Which brings us to this special issue of the *Journal of Gay & Lesbian Psychotherapy*. In this Special Issue of the publication, we profile the evolving status of mental health services in the public sector for LGBT individuals, and the expanding role of clinicians, administrators, and mental health advocates who are contributing to the establishment and provision of these services in both traditional and nontraditional settings.

The papers are organized to provide readers with an overview of issues in this area, to give a perspective on developments at the federal and state levels, to characterize some existing clinical programs in the public sector, to offer examples of case material that illustrate concerns that arise for clinicians working with LGBT people in public psychiatry, and in two interviews, to discern the thoughts, experience, and opinions of leaders in the field.

The first article, "Sexual Minorities and Mental Health: The Need for a Public Health Response," addresses the provision of mental health services to sexual minorities in the United States through the history of funding and programming at the federal level. Based on their review, Karina Uldall, MD, and Nancy Palmer, PhD, argue for the need to develop a coordinated federal initiative to address the mental health needs of the LGBT community. Dr. Uldall is Associate Professor in the Department of Psychiatry and Behavioral Sciences at the University of Washington, and is Attending Psychiatrist with the University of Washington Medical Center and Harborview Medical Center. She is the Principal Investigator for research on prevention efforts with HIV positive individuals, and has previously authored numerous papers and book chapters. Dr. Palmer's doctorate is in the history of sexuality. She has studied the social and cultural construction of sexuality. Currently, she is working in the area of sexually transmitted diseases and HIV behavioral research in Seattle, WA.

In the next article, entitled "Lesbian, Gay, Bisexual, and Transgender People Receiving Services in the Public Mental Health System: Raising Issues" Alicia Lucksted, PhD, applies survey research methods to ascertain a range of views and concerns that highlight questions and themes important to the welfare of LGBT people receiving public/community mental health services. She surveys archival documents, including published and unpublished literature, and through the personal testimony of key informants, such as mental health providers and those who use mental health services, begins to delineate a picture of the essential issues and questions that distinguish this area of clinical practice. Dr. Lucksted is a clinical-community psychologist in the Department of Psychiatry at the University of Maryland in the Center for Mental Health Services Research. Her work has focused on the views of those who use mental health services in evaluation and academic research regarding the U.S. public mental health system, with particular emphasis on the issues and welfare of LGBT people receiving mental health services.

In "Advocating for Health and Human Services: The New York Experience," Sheila A. Healy, MPA, describes how LGBT organizations in New York State organized to gain public funding for mental health and other human services. She documents how a new advocacy strategy was pioneered in New York State, by consolidating LGBT human service organizations into a statewide network that subsequently partnered with New York's political advocacy organization, the Empire State Pride Agenda (ESPA). This approach created a powerful entity that gained state recognition and public funding for LGBT social service and mental health programs. Ms. Healy was the Program Director of the Empire State Pride Agenda Foundation, the non-partisan education, research, and advocacy arm of ESPA. In 2004, she became the Executive Director of the National Association of Lesbian, Gay, Bisexual and Transgender Community Centers in Washington, DC.

The next paper, by Ronald E. Hellman, MD, and Eileen Klein, PhD, is entitled "A Program for Lesbian, Gay, Bisexual, and Transgender Individuals with Major Mental Illness." They describe how a culturally sensitive program for LGBT people with major mental illness was developed in New York State's largest community mental health center. Dr. Hellman is Director of the program and has been active in the LGBT community for over 30 years. Dr. Klein is Adjunct Professor in the School of Social Work at NYU, and is a Chief of Service at South Beach Psychiatric Center in New York City.

The article by Medeiros, Seehaus, Elliott, and Melaney entitled "Providing Mental Health Services for GLBT Teens in a Community Adolescent Health Clinic," describes the rationale for encompassing mental health care for sexual minority teens within a medical clinic setting. They describe how LGBT teenagers, and adolescents questioning their sexual identity, are evaluated and referred to specialized groups provided to help them navigate through issues particular to LGBT adolescents as they come to terms with their sexual minority status. Daniel Medeiros, MD, is currently directing an adolescent chemical dependency day program, and day program for teens with emotional issues at St. Luke's Roosevelt Hospital Center in New York City. This paper is based upon his work at the Mt. Sinai Adolescent Health Center (MSAHC) in New York, where he directed mental health services for five years. Mavis Seehaus, CSW, is the Supervisor of the Primary Care Social Work Program and the Health Education Program at MSAHC. Jennifer Elliot, CSW, works with HIV-affected adolescents in the Ryan White/Project Impact program at MSAHC. Adam Melaney, CSW, also works in the Ryan White program.

Daniel Garza, MD, is Assistant Clinical Professor of Psychiatry at Mount Sinai Medical Center in New York. He currently directs the Assisted Outpatient Treatment Program at Elmhurst Hospital Center, is a volunteer with Disaster Psychiatry Outreach, and is a consulting psychiatrist with the Callen-Lorde Community Health Center. In his article, "The Community Health Project," he recounts the development of the Callen-Lorde Health Center in New York City, from its origins as a small, volunteer agency, the Community Health Project, to a multi-million dollar health care facility. He describes the program's growth in the provision of comprehensive health care services for the LGBT community in New York City, and the concurrent evolution of mental health services in this unique medical setting.

In "Group Psychotherapy for HIV-Positive Veterans in a Veterans Administration Clinic," Michael Rankin, MD, describes the challenges encountered while running a psychotherapy group for HIV positive veterans in a VA clinic during the mid-1980s, a time of homophobia and AIDS phobia in the federal public health system. Dr. Rankin is former Commissioner of Mental Health in Arkansas from 1978-1980 and is currently Clinical Professor of Psychiatry and Behavioral Sciences at the George Washington University Medical School in Washington, DC. From 1993-2000, he was a member of the President's Advisory Council on HIV and AIDS.

Michael C. Singer, in "Being Gay and Mentally Ill: The Case Study of a Gay Man with Schizophrenia Treated at a Community Mental Health Facility," describes his clinical work with a gay man diagnosed with schizophrenia, applying principles from psychodynamic and cultural psychiatry in a mainstream community mental health setting. Dr. Singer is currently on the faculty in the Department of Psychology at Hunter College and in private practice, following his appointment as Clinical Assistant Instructor in the Department of Psychiatry at Downstate Medical Center in Brooklyn, New York.

In his article "Treatment of a Transgender Client with Schizophrenia in a Public Psychiatric Milieu: A Case Study by a Student Therapist," Noel R. Garrett discusses the complex challenges that arose while in training to be a psychologist during his clinical experience in a community mental health center. There, he worked with a transgender patient diagnosed with major mental illness. Noel R. Garrett has a Master of Arts in Psychology from the New School University in New York, and is a Doctoral candidate in Clinical Psychology at the New School.

This issue concludes with two interviews. They were conducted with Francis G. Lu, MD and Barbara E. Warren, PsyD, both individuals of exceptional character and stamina, who established two of the largest public sector mental health programs for LGBT people in the United States. Both are heterosexual, and both have been strong allies of the LGBT community. Over many years, they have tirelessly advocated for sensitive and culturally relevant mental health services to overcome the disparities that exist for underserved sexual minorities with mental health issues. The interviews profile how they became involved with LGBT issues and then went on to develop major public sector LGBT programs. Their experience and thoughts should provide important insights for anyone interested in public mental health services for sexual minorities.

Ronald E. Hellman, MD
Jack Drescher, MD

NOTE

1. This study utilized more precise definitions of homosexuality and heterosexuality, inquiring about individual desire, behavior, and identity, and obtained a carefully stratified representative sampling of the general population. The total number of persons reporting at least one of the components of homosexuality was only 293 in a total sample of 3159, 150 of 1749 women and 143 of 1410 men. Consequently, the number of persons reporting same-sex desire, behavior, and identity in specific age groups, in different geographic locations, and in other demographic categories was rather small. This study showed that of the total sample, 1.3% of the women and 2.7% of the men participated in same-sex sexual behavior during the preceding year, and 4.1% of women and 4.9% of men had done so since age 18; 7.5% of women and 7.7% of men reported the presence of sexual desire for someone of the same sex; and 1.4% of the women and 2.8% of the men reported a homosexual or bisexual identity. These figures varied considerably across groups based on age, marital status, education, religion, race, and place of residence.

REFERENCES

Alexander, F.G. & Selesnick, S.T. (1966), *The History of Psychiatry: An Evaluation of Psychiatric Thought and Practice from Prehistoric Times to the Present*. New York: Harper & Row.

Altman, D. (1982), *The Homosexualization of America*. New York: St. Martin's Press.

Bayer, R. (1981), *Homosexuality and American Psychiatry: The Politics of Diagnosis*. New York: Basic Books.

Bieber, I., Dain, H., Dince, P., Drellich, M., Grand, H., Gundlach, R., Kremer, M., Rifkin, A., Wilbur, C. & Bieber, T. (1962), *Homosexuality: A Psychoanalytic Study*. New York: Basic Books.

Drescher, J. (2003), An interview with Robert L. Spitzer, MD. *J. Gay & Lesbian Psychotherapy*, 7(3):97-11.

Foucault, M. (1978), *The History of Sexuality, Volume I, An Introduction*. Originally published as *Histoire de la sexualité 1: La volonté de savoir* (Paris: Gallimard). New York: Vintage, 1980.

Grob, G.N. (1994), The history of the asylum revisited: Personal reflections. In: *Discovering the History of Psychiatry*, eds. M.S. Micale & R. Porter. Oxford: Oxford University Press, 260-281.

Group for the Advancement of Psychiatry (2000), *Homosexuality and the Mental Health Professions: The Impact of Bias*. Hillsdale, NJ: The Analytic Press.

Hire, R.O. (2002), An interview with Robert Jean Campbell III, MD. *J. Gay & Lesbian Psychotherapy*, 6(3): 81-96.

Johnsgard, K. & Schumacher, R. (1970), The experience of intimacy in group psychotherapy with male homosexuals. *Psychotherapy: Theory, Research & Practice*, 7:173-176.

Katz, J. (1983), *Gay/Lesbian Almanac*. New York: Carroll & Graf Publishers, Inc.

Kent, J.J. & Gibson, R.W. (1992), Governmental legislation and regulation. In: *Textbook of Administrative Psychiatry*, ed. J.A. Talbott, R.E. Hales & S.L. Keill. Washington, DC: American Psychiatric Press, pp. 207-250.

Kinsey, A., Pomeroy, W. & Martin, C. (1948), *Sexual Behavior in the Human Male*. Philadelphia, PA: Saunders.

Kinsey, A., Pomeroy, W., Martin, C. & Gebhard, P. (1953), *Sexual Behavior in the Human Female*. Philadelphia, PA: Saunders.

Kuhn, T. (1972), *The Structure of Scientific Revolutions. Second Edition*, Chicago, IL: The University of Chicago Press.

Laumann, E.O., Gagnon, J.H., Michael, R.T. & Michaels, S, (1994), *The Social Organization of Sexuality: Sexual Practices in the United States*. Chicago: University of Chicago Press.

McCarn, S. (1999), Meeting the mental health needs of gay, lesbian, bisexual, and transgender persons. *Cultural Diversity Series*. National Technical Assistance Center for State Mental Health Planning, 2, August.

Mechanic, D. (2003), Managing behavioral health in medicaid. Editorial, *N. Engl. J. Med.*, 348: 1914.

Mora, G. (1975), Historical and theoretical trends in psychiatry. In: *Comprehensive Textbook of Psychiatry/II*, eds. A.M. Freedman, H.I. Kaplan & B. J. Sadock. Baltimore: The Williams & Wilkins Co., pp. 1-75.

National Association of State Mental Health Program Directors (2000), *Position Statement on Culturally Competent and Linguistically Appropriate Mental Health Services*. MASMHPD Website (*http://www.nasmhpd.org/linguist.htm*), June.

Rosario, V.A. (2003), An interview with Judd Marmor, MD. *J. Gay & Lesbian Psychotherapy*, 7(4):23-34.

Sbordone, A.J. (2003), An interview with Charles Silverstein, PhD. *J. Gay & Lesbian Psychotherapy*, 7(4):49-61.

Scasta, D.L. (2002), John E. Fryer, MD, and the Dr. H. Anonymous episode. *J. Gay & Lesbian Psychotherapy*, 6(4):73-84.

Silverstein, C. (1995), *Gays, Lesbians, and Their Therapists: Studies in Psychotherapy*. New York: W.W. Norton.

Talbott, J.A. & Hales, R.E. (2001), *Textbook of Administrative Psychiatry: New Concepts for a Changing Behavioral Health System*. Washington, DC: American Psychiatric Press.

Thompson, M., ed. (1994), *Long Road to Freedom: The Advocate History of the Gay and Lesbian Movement*. New York: St. Martin's Press.

Weinberg, M.S. & Bell, A.P. (1972), *Homosexuality: An Annotated Bibliography*. New York: Harper & Row.

Sexual Minorities and Mental Health: The Need for a Public Health Response

Karina K. Uldall, MD, MPH
Nancy B. Palmer, PhD

SUMMARY. This paper outlines the public mental health response to sexual minorities in the United States. Information from the academic literature, federal and state initiatives, and the work of the organized lesbian, gay, bisexual and transgender (LGBT) communities is placed in an historical context of mental health attitudes toward homosexuality. In addition to recommendations for future directions in research and treatment, the authors present an argument for establishing a coordinated federal initiative to address some of the unique mental health needs of the LGBT community. *[Article copies available for a fee from The Haworth Document Delivery Service: 1-800-HAWORTH. E-mail address: <docdelivery@ haworthpress.com> Website: <http://www.HaworthPress.com> © 2004 by The Haworth Press, Inc. All rights reserved.]*

KEYWORDS. Bisexual, federal, gay, government, homosexuality, lesbian, mental health, public health, public psychiatry, sexual minorities, sexual orientation, transgender

---

Karina K. Uldall is affiliated with the Department of Psychiatry, University of Washington School of Medicine, Seattle, WA.

Nancy B. Palmer is affiliated with the Center for Health Training, Seattle, WA.

Address correspondence to: Karina K. Uldall, MD, MPH, 901 Boren Avenue, Suite 900, Seattle, WA 98104 (E-mail: keegan@u.washington.edu).

[Haworth co-indexing entry note]: "Sexual Minorities and Mental Health: The Need for a Public Health Response." Uldall, Karina K., and Nancy B. Palmer. Co-published simultaneously in *Journal of Gay & Lesbian Psychotherapy* (The Haworth Medical Press, an imprint of The Haworth Press, Inc.) Vol. 8, No. 3/4, 2004, pp. 11-24; and: *Handbook of LGBT Issues in Community Mental Health* (ed: Ronald E. Hellman, and Jack Drescher) The Haworth Medical Press, an imprint of The Haworth Press, Inc., 2004, pp. 11-24. Single or multiple copies of this article are available for a fee from The Haworth Document Delivery Service [1-800-HAWORTH, 9:00 a.m. - 5:00 p.m. (EST). E-mail address: docdelivery@haworthpress.com].

INTRODUCTION

Mentally ill lesbian, gay, bisexual and transgender (LGBT) individuals face a dual stigma in society: they are frequently discriminated against by virtue of their health issues, as well as their sexual orientation and gender identity. The environment in which GLBT individuals seek health care is further complicated by historical events, particularly the gay movement's history of activism against the mental health profession's historical categorization of homosexuality as a mental illness. In the public health arena, efforts to normalize and to de-stigmatize sexual orientation and gender identity exist alongside attempts to provide effective care for mentally ill LGBT individuals.

This paper outlines the public health response to sexual minorities in the U.S. Due to an absence of literature on sexual minorities and mental health, the paper focuses on funding and programming at the federal level. It highlights some of the complications and outcomes of federal efforts to address the mental health needs of LGBT people. It concludes with an argument for a coordinated federal initiative to begin to address some of the unique mental health needs of the LGBT community.

HISTORICAL BACKGROUND

Since the 19th century, there were those in the medical profession who classified homosexuality as a mental disorder (Krafft-Ebing, 1886). Until 1973, the American Psychiatric Association's (APA) classification of homosexuality as a mental disorder (American Psychiatric Association, 1952 and 1968) contributed to an atmosphere of stigmatization and marginalization of the LGBT population. As a result, the APA's diagnostic manual also provided a focal point for resistance and gay activism (Bayer, 1981). However, drawing upon the scientific work of Kinsey (Kinsey, Pomeroy and Martin, 1948; Kinsey et al., 1953), Ford and Beach (1951), Hooker (1957), and Marmor (1965), activists argued to the APA that homosexuals are as well adjusted as heterosexuals. The APA ultimately removed homosexuality from its list of mental disorders in 1973 (Krajeski, 1996; Hire, 2002; Scasta, 2002; Drescher, 2003; Rosario, 2003; Sbordone, 2003).

In subsequent position statements adopted by the APA, discrimination based on sexual orientation has been consistently deplored (American Psychiatric Association, 1973, 1984, 1988, 1990, 1991, & 1992). More recently, the inclusion of sexual orientation in the organization's definition of cultural diversity (1999), and its stance opposing "reparative" or "conversion" therapy aimed at changing one's sexual orientation (1998 and 2000a), have both exemplified efforts to decrease stigma aimed at LGBT individuals. Most recently, the APA stated its organizational support for same-sex unions (2000b) and for the adoption/co-parenting of children by same-sex couples (2002). Since 1973, each step made by the APA, the leading professional organization for psychiatrists in the United States, has effectively contributed to the de-marginalization and de-stigmatization of LGBT individuals in the U.S. [1]

FEDERAL AND STATE RESPONSE TO SEXUAL MINORITIES AND MENTAL HEALTH

Since the declassification of homosexuality as a mental illness, there has been little public attention to the mental health needs of sexual minorities. What was once categorized as a mental illness has become a virtually invisible issue in the public mental health arena. The presence or absence of mental health research, and subsequently of treatment, focused on LGBT individuals in the public sector has mirrored the prevailing cultural and sociopolitical climate in the United States. Significantly, there is no agency within the Department of Health infrastructure that is mandated to promote research or policy studies on LGBT health. Without a coordinating agency, federal efforts in this area are episodic and lack a clear public health agenda. For example, national surveys on the prevalence of mental illness, such as the Epidemiologic Catchment Area Study (Robins and Regier, 1991) and the National Comorbidity Study (Kessler et al., 1994), did not contain questions regarding sexual orientation. The subsequent lack of population-based information on which to base policy or to formulate research questions compromises the articulation of a public mental health agenda for the LGBT population.

The experience of the National Association of State Mental Health Program Directors is instructive on this point. The National Association included sexual orientation among its list of characteristics to define culturally competent mental health services in June 2000. However, three years later, this position statement has not been implemented across the nation. The statement identifies the need to develop and disseminate information and technical assistance, provide forums for state and national dialogues, and develop research, education, training and performance-based initiatives on effective provision of culturally competent mental health services, including services to LGBT populations. Specific funding and a detailed plan to implement this effort remain unclear. Further, efforts aimed at the sexual minority community can easily be lost in states with more visible culturally diverse populations based on race, ethnicity, religion, language or national origin. Limited State resources limit the initiatives aimed at sexual minority mental health.

Throughout most of the twentieth century, LGBT mental health issues have not been targeted by federal initiatives, funding agencies, or academics, with the exception of those few individuals who have been personally motivated to pursue this area of research. Review of the Federal Register on-line database from 1995 through 2002 revealed very few funding opportunities specific to the area of homosexuality, sexual minority or lesbian/gay and mental health (Federal Register, 1995-2002). One exception to this trend can be seen in the federal response to the advent of HIV/AIDS in the 1980s. The groundswell of community activism around this disease forced federal agencies, researchers and treatment providers to address issues specific to at least one segment of the sexual minority population–gay men. The resources allocated to the research and treatment of HIV/AIDS have typically included monies for mental health and substance abuse (Federal Register, 1995-2002). More recently, however, funding opportunities focused on HIV have followed trends in the HIV epidemic, now targeting people of color and youth in place of sexual minorities.

It has sometimes been the case that even if a report on the topic of LGBT people and mental health has been researched, written and published, the report has not been reproduced or disseminated in any way, so that it ends up having little or no impact. For example, in 1999 the Institute of Medicine published a landmark report entitled *Lesbian Health: Current Assessment and Directions for the Future* (Solarz, 1999). Mental health and substance abuse were two areas addressed specifically by this effort. Resiliency/Health effects of homophobia, service delivery and access to services were also addressed. Even though the report was published, the ability to implement the report without specific funding initiatives remains uncertain.

The U.S. Surgeon General published *Mental Health: A Report of the Surgeon General* in 1999 (U.S. Department of Health and Human Services, 1999). Themes of the U.S. Surgeon General's Report include: mental health and mental illness require the broad focus of a public health approach; mental health and mental illness are points on a continuum; and stigma is a major obstacle preventing people from getting help.

This report was followed by the supplement entitled *Mental Health: Culture, Race, Ethnicity* (U.S. Department of Health and Human Services, 2000a). The Supplement was written to address mental health disparities of racial and ethnic minorities. Specific goals of the Supplement include: helping readers to understand the nature and extent of mental health disparities; to present evidence on the need for mental health services and the provision of services to meet those needs; to document promising directions toward the elimination of mental health disparities and the promotion of mental health.

Both of these documents discussed the stigma of mental illness and the need to address health disparities in accessing mental health services. Although LGBT populations were not addressed directly in the Supplement, one could argue that many of the conclusions of the Supplement apply to LGBT individuals. Not specifying sexual minorities, however, could also have important implications in terms of lack of funding for research and treatment targeting LGBT populations.

The Substance Abuse and Mental Health Services Administration (SAMSHA), Center for Mental Health Services, is one federal agency that has attempted to address the specific needs of LGBT individuals. A monograph on the needs of consumers who identified as LGBT was developed in 1999, as a result of the lack of published material on this topic. According to the author, Alicia Lucksted, however, the monograph became ensnarled in the bureaucratic process. Although it was heavily researched and written with the help of a professional writer hired by SAMSHA, the latter never published it and ownership reverted back to the author.[2]

The lack of a coordinated federal response to LGBT mental health issues can result in inconsistent dissemination efforts. For example, at the same time that the SAMSHA monograph on the needs of LGBT consumers was effectively shelved, its author noted that a substance use report addressing a provider's introduction to substance abuse in LGBT people was produced and disseminated by SAMHSA (personal communication with A. Lucksted, 3/2003). Clearly, the lack of a coordinated federal response to LGBT issues makes the dissemination and implementation of any effort uneven and unpredictable.

In March of 2001, the *Healthy People 2010 Companion Document for LGBT Health* was released. This paper was a collaborative effort on the part of the Gay and Lesbian Medical Association (GLMA), LGBT health experts and the National Coalition for LGBT Health. Mental health/mental disorders and substance abuse were two of the focus areas addressed, in keeping with the twelve focus areas of the federal blueprint for public health, *Healthy People 2010* (U.S. Department of Health and Human Services, 2000b). Although the stated goal of *Healthy People 2010* is to eliminate health disparities in America, the Department of Health and Human Services did not fund the dissemination of the companion document.[3] In the end, Congress was presented with a strategic plan for funding submitted by the Department of Health and Human Services that only included gender, race/ethnicity, education/income, disability and geographic location. Sexual orientation was completely omitted from the list of disparities to be addressed, which has grave implications in terms of federal funding priorities.

LITERATURE REVIEW

Searches of the academic literature have produced very little in the area of LGBT mental health research and treatment (Oetjen and Rothblum, 2000; Ayala and Coleman, 2000; Cochran and Mays, 2000a, b; Herek, Gillis and Cogan, 1999; Fergusson, Horwood and Beautrais, 1999; Garofalo et al., 1998, 1999; Remafedi et al., 1998; Faulkner and Cranston, 1998; Sorensen and

Roberts, 1997; Brown et al., 1996; Meyer, 1995; Meyer and Dean, 1995, 1998). Papers addressing the care of LGBT populations in the public sector appear to be non-existent. A perhaps unintended effect of a lack of funding targeting LGBT mental health issues is that the absence of funding can lead to an absence of research on mental health treatment options for LGBT people. Even if individual researchers are personally interested in pursuing research in this area, their work will necessarily be constrained by a lack of funding.

Cochran and Mays (2000b) attempted to define the relationship between psychiatric illness, including addictive disorders, and sexual orientation in a sample of the U.S. population. Their work was impeded by sampling problems, however, which adversely affects the ability to generalize these findings to the larger LGBT population. Other population-based studies have focused predominantly on youth (Faulkner and Cranston, 1998; Garofalo et al., 1998, 1999).

Of the few studies that have been conducted on the LGBT population and mental health, most publications have focused on the prevalence of mood disorders, anxiety disorders and suicide attempts among gay men (Cochran and Mays, 2000a; Meyer, 1995; Meyer and Dean, 1995,1998; Fergusson, Horwood and Beautrais,1999; Remafedi, Farrow and Deischer,1991; Remafedi et al., 1998; Rotheram-Borus, Hunter and Rosario, 1994; Williams et al., 1991; Ross, 1990; Schneider, Farberow and Kruks,1989; Rich et al., 1986). The National Lesbian Health Care Survey (Bradford, Ryan and Rothblum, 1994) focused on depression. Other studies of lesbians have addressed factors cited in the general literature on women and depression, such as relationship status and social support (Oetjen and Rothblum,, 2000; Ayala and Coleman, 2000). While some studies involving transgender persons have suggested a higher frequency of personality disorders and psychoses among that population (Derogatis, Meyer and Vazquez, 1978; Dixen et al., 1984; Beatrice, 1985; Hartmann, Becker and Rueffer-Hesse,1997), more recent publications have countered these findings (Cole et al., 1997; Brown et al., 1996).

Several papers have demonstrated the importance of tailoring systems of care providing mental health treatment, including prevention programs, to address specific needs of the LGBT population. In 1996, the Council on Scientific Affairs of the American Medical Association published a paper on the health care needs of gay men and lesbians that emphasized the need to understand patterns of and risk factors for mental disorders among LGBT individuals (Council on Scientific Affairs, 1996). One year later, the Boston Lesbian Health Project published data regarding lesbian use of and satisfaction with mental health services (Sorensen and Roberts, 1997). Other studies have documented the dissatisfaction among LGBT recipients of mental health services (Garnets et al., 1991; Liddle, 1996). Still others have argued that transgender persons are a particularly vulnerable and underserved population in the U.S.

medical system, due to the prejudice against them that is pervasive in U.S. medicine (Lawrence et al., 1996). As in other sectors of society, transgender does not fit neatly into one gender category or another, which has ramifications within the medical establishment.

RECOMMENDATIONS FOR THE FUTURE

Epidemiology

The need for good data on the incidence and prevalence of mental disorders, including addictive disorders, among LGBT individuals is fundamental to future research and treatment endeavors. No federal survey currently asks for information about sexual orientation linked to mental health issues. Without this information, policy makers, researchers and treatment providers cannot grasp the magnitude or quality of mental illness among the LGBT population. Sexual orientation and gender identity data should be included in national studies and surveillance systems.

Prevention

Prevention is defined as decreasing the risk or delaying the onset of a mental disorder. For example, the prevention of substance abuse among LGBT youth lends itself to intervention, since it is known that mental health problems in children and adolescents precede the onset of substance abuse problems by several years (Garofalo, 1998).

Identification and promotion of resiliency factors is central to any mental health prevention effort. LGBT persons, often facing stressful situations throughout their lives as a result of their sexual minority status, are potential prototypes of resiliency (Levy, 1992; Clements et al., 1999; Kennedy, 2000). This means that studies in this area among LGBT individuals could additionally benefit health care in populations other than the sexual minority population.

Co-Occurring Mental Disorders and Substance Abuse

Due to the association of substance abuse and dependence with other mental disorders and the apparent frequency of substance abuse/dependence among LGBT populations (Chesney, Barrett and Stall,1998; DuRant, Krowchuk and Sinal, 1998; Flavin, Franklin and Frances, 1996; Kruks, 1991; McKirnan and Peterson, 1989; Glaus, 1988), interventions addressing the needs of individuals with co-occurring disorders require further study. The content, timing and order of interventions for LGBT dually diagnosed persons have not been addressed to date.

Treatment Across the Lifespan

Specific topics for interventions in this area include reduction in the rate of suicide attempts among LGBT youth, adults and elders; addressing self-esteem and body image in the context of eating disorders among gay youth; integrating LGBT psychiatric care, including addiction treatment, into primary care settings; and integrating LGBT youth psychiatric care into public sector agencies that serve youth, e.g., schools.

Consumer/Family Involvement

The role of mentally ill LGBT persons and their families in the development of services, prevention of discrimination towards individuals with mental disorders, and promotion of recovery cannot be underestimated. Both individuals and systems of care benefit from active involvement of members of the target population in the design, implementation and evaluation of interventions. Currently funded mental health consumer groups should consistently include sexual orientation and gender identity among the special populations served.

Education and Training

Improving primary care and mental health providers' ability to treat LGBT individuals effectively and in a culturally competent manner must receive financial and administrative support at post-graduate schools across the nation. Continuing education opportunities in LGBT mental health care for those providers already working should be a requirement for licensing and certification. Education and training activities must also include information about community resources and referrals appropriate for the LGBT population. Evaluation of education and training programs is essential to insure the success of these efforts.

Political Strategies

There are many LGBT institutions and organizations that have been working for years on issues unique to LGBT populations, from the National Gay and Lesbian Task Force (NGLTF), an early advocate of efforts to declassify homosexuality as a mental illness, to the Gay and Lesbian Medical Association (GLMA) which assisted in the development of the LGBT companion document to *Healthy People 2010*. Hundreds of community-based organizations

(CBOs) across the U.S., such as the Los Angeles Gay and Lesbian Community Center and the New York Gay and Lesbian Community Center, have implemented programs addressing LGBT issues including mental health and substance abuse. What is lacking is a way to link LGBT program directors and policy advisors who are already working in this area to some coordinated, sustained, and consistent mechanism for implementation and dissemination at the federal and state level.

CONCLUSION

Without a federal agency with a clear mandate to address the mental health issues associated with the lesbian, gay, bisexual and transgender populations, this segment of U.S. society will remain vulnerable. States and local governments cannot be relied on to address emerging LGBT mental health issues in a consistent or even minimally efficient manner without federal leadership. Despite the existence of professional organizations that have outlined, and will continue to detail, various components of a national response to LGBT mental health, the absence of the necessary federal infrastructure and coordinated funding opportunities impedes the successful implementation and dissemination of these ideas and initiatives. It is time to articulate and implement a unified national agenda to address LGBT mental health issues.

NOTES

1. One caveat to this narrative is that transgender individuals maintain an even more complicated relationship to the psychiatric profession than gay, lesbian or bisexual individuals at this time. While homosexual identity became defined by the 1960s as largely divorced from gender and focused instead on sexual object choice (Kennedy, 1993), the definition of transgender is currently still framed by ideas about gender. As such, it is a sexual minority identity that is subject to classification by the psychiatric (and other) communities. For example, the *Diagnostic and Statistical Manual of Mental Disorders, Fourth Edition* (American Psychiatric Association, 1994), contains four diagnostic categories potentially applicable to transgender persons: gender identity disorder in adolescents and adults; gender identity disorder in children; gender identity disorder not otherwise specified; and transvestic fetishism. While diagnosis of these disorders technically requires evidence of distress or functional impairment (other than that due to societal prejudice based on perceived social deviance), the very process of categorization, as seen in the history of homosexuality and mental illness, can function to allow mental health providers and others to view transgender individuals as psychiatrically ill.

2. After two years, the monograph was not approved by the federal clearance process, and the author could not get a definitive response as to why. Whether or not the

federal decision was the result of politics and the change in administration, systemic homophobia, a simple case of bureaucratic disorganization, or some combination of these, was never clear to the author (personal communication with A. Lucksted, 3/2003).

3. One member of GLMA who worked on this document at the time, Darren Carter, recalls that people were focused on the publication of the document, and realized only as an afterthought that there was no funding for dissemination (personal communication with D. Carter, 3/2003).

REFERENCES

American Psychiatric Association (1952), *Diagnostic and Statistical Manual of Mental Disorders*. Washington, DC: American Psychiatric Association.

American Psychiatric Association (1968), *Diagnostic and Statistical Manual of Mental Disorders, Second Edition*. Washington, DC: American Psychiatric Association.

American Psychiatric Association (1973), *Homosexuality and Civil Rights*. American Psychiatric Association Website (www.psych.org/libr_publ/position.htm).

American Psychiatric Association (1980), *Diagnostic and Statistical Manual of Mental Disorders, Third Edition*. Washington, DC: American Psychiatric Press.

American Psychiatric Association (1984), *Homosexual Issues Concerning the Military*. American Psychiatric Association Website (www.psych.org/libr_publ/position.htm).

American Psychiatric Association (1988), *Statement on Discrimination Based on Gender or Sexual Orientation*. American Psychiatric Association Website (www.psych.org/libr_publ/position.htm).

American Psychiatric Association (1990), *Homosexuality and the Armed Services*. American Psychiatric Association Website (www.psych.org/libr_publ/position.htm).

American Psychiatric Association (1991), *Homosexuality and the Immigration and Naturalization Service*. American Psychiatric Association Website (www.psych.org/libr_publ/position.htm).

American Psychiatric Association (1992), *Homosexuality*. American Psychiatric Association Website (www.psych.org/libr_publ/position.htm).

American Psychiatric Association (1994), *Diagnostic and Statistical Manual of Mental Disorders, Fourth Edition*. Washington, DC: American Psychiatric Association.

American Psychiatric Association (1998), *Psychiatric Treatment and Sexual Orientation*. American Psychiatric Association Website (www.psych.org/libr_publ/position.htm).

American Psychiatric Association (1999), *Diversity*. American Psychiatric Association Website (www.psych.org/libr_publ/position.htm).

American Psychiatric Association (2000a), *Therapies Focused on Attempts to Change Sexual Orientation ("Reparative" or Conversion Therapies)*. American Psychiatric Association Website (www.psych.org/libr_publ/position.htm).

American Psychiatric Association (2000b), *Same Sex Unions*. American Psychiatric Association Website (www.psych.org/libr_publ/position.htm).

American Psychiatric Association (2002), *Adoption and Co-Parenting of Children by Same-Sex Couples*. American Psychiatric Association Website (www.psych.org/libr_publ/position.htm).

Ayala, J., & Coleman, H. (2000), Predictors of depression among lesbian women. *J. Lesbian Studies*, 4:71-86.

Bayer, R. (1981), *Homosexuality and American Psychiatry: The Politics of Diagnosis.* New York: Basic Books.

Beatrice, J. (1985), A psychological comparison of heterosexuals, transvestites, preoperative transsexuals, and postoperative transsexuals. *J. Nervous & Mental Disorders*, 173:358-365.

Bradford, J., Ryan, C., & Rothblum, E.D. (1994), National Lesbian Health Care Survey: Implications for mental health care. *J. Consulting & Clinical Psychology*, 52:228-242.

Brown, G.R., Wise, T.N., Costa, P.T. Jr., Herbst, J.H., Fagan, P.J. & Schmidt, C.W. Jr. (1996), Personality characteristics and sexual functioning of 199 cross-dressing men. *J. Nervous & Mental Disorders*, 184:265-273.

Chauncey, G. (1994), *Gay New York: Gender, Urban Culture and the Making of the Gay Male World 1890-1940.* New York, NY: Basic Books.

Chesney, M.A., Barrett, D.C., & Stall, R. (1998), Histories of substance use and risk behavior: Precursors to HIV seroconversion in homosexual men. *American J. of Public Health*, 88:113-116.

Clements, K., Wilkinson, W., Kitano, K., & Marx, R. (1999), Prevention and health service needs of the transgender community in San Francisco. *International J. Transgenderism*, 3.

Cochran, S.D., & Mays V.M. (2000a), Lifetime prevalence of suicide symptoms and affective disorders among men reporting same-sex sexual partners: Results from NHANES III. *American J. Public Health*, 90:573-578.

Cochran, S.D. & Mays, V.M. (2000b), Relation between psychiatric syndromes and behaviorally defined sexual orientation in a sample of the US population. *American J. Epidemiology*, 151:516-523.

Cole, C., O'Boyle, M., Emory, L., & Meyer, W. (1997), Co-morbidity of gender dysphoria and other major psychiatric diagnoses. *Archives Sexual Behavior*, 26: 13-26.

Council on Scientific Affairs, American Medical Association (1996), Health care needs of gay men and lesbians in the United States. *J. American Medical Association*, 275:1354-1359.

Derogatis, L., Meyer, J. & Vazquez, N. (1978), A psychological profile of the transsexual. I. The male. *J. Nervous & Mental Disorders*, 166:234-254.

Dixen, J.M., Maddever, H., Van Maasden, J. & Edwards, P.W. (1984), Psychosocial characteristics of applicants evaluated for surgical gender reassignment. *Archives Sexual Behavior*, 13:269-277.

Drescher, J. (2003), An interview with Robert L. Spitzer, MD. *J. Gay & Lesbian Psychotherapy*, 7(3):97-111.

DuRant, R.H., Krowchuk, D.P. & Sinal, S.H. (1998), Victimization, use of violence, and drug use at school among male adolescents who engage in same-sex sexual behavior. *J. Pediatrics*, 133:113-118.

Faulkner, A.H. & Cranston, K. (1998), Correlates of same-sex sexual behavior in a random sample of Massachusetts high school students. *American J. Public Health*, 88:262-266.

Federal Register (1995-2002), Federal Register Website (http://frwebgate3.access. gpo.gov/).

Fergusson, D.M., Horwood, L.J. & Beautrais, A.L. (1999), Is sexual orientation related to mental health problems and suicidality in young people? *Archives General Psychiatry,* 56:876-880.

Flavin, D.K., Frankin, E.J. & Frances, R.J. (1996), Acquired immune deficiency syndrome (AIDS) and suicidal behavior in alcohol-dependent homosexual men. *American J. Psychiatry,* 143:1440-1442.

Ford, C. & Beach, F. (1951), *Patterns of Sexual Behavior.* New York: Harper.

Garnets, L., Hancock, K.A., Cochran, S.D., Goodchilds, J. & Peplau, L.A. (1991), Issues in psychotherapy with lesbians and gay men: A survey of psychologists. *American Psychologist,* 46:964-972.

Garofalo, R., Wolf, R.C., Kessel, S., Palfrey, S.J. & Durant, R.H. (1998), The association between health risk behaviors and sexual orientation among a school-based sample of adolescents. *Pediatrics,* 101:895-902.

Garofalo, R., Wolf, R.C., Wissow, L.S., Woods, E.R. & Goodman, E. (1999), Sexual orientation and risk of suicide attempts among a representative sample of youth. *Archives Pediatric & Adolescent Medicine,* 153:487-493.

Glaus, O. (1988), Alcoholism, chemical dependency, and the lesbian client. *Women & Therapy,* 8:131-144.

Hartmann, U., Becker, H. & Rueffer-Hesse, C. (1997), Self and gender: Narcissistic pathology and personality factors in gender dysphoric patients: Preliminary results of a prospective study. *International Journal Transgenderism,* 1. International Journal of Transgenderism Website (www.symposion.com/itj/itjc0103.htm).

Herek, G.M., Gillis, J.R. & Cogan, J.C. (1999), Psychological sequelae of hate-crime victimization among lesbian, gay, and bisexual adults. *J. Consulting & Clinical Psychology,* 67:945-951.

Hire, R.O. (2002), An interview with Robert Jean Campbell III, MD. *J. Gay & Lesbian Psychotherapy,* 6(3):81-96.

Hooker, E. (1957), The adjustment of the male overt homosexual. *J. Projective Technique,* 21:18-31.

Kennedy, N.J. (2000), Preventing and treating behavioral health problems in gay America: Traversing life and culture. Position paper for Lesbian, Gay, Bisexual and Transgender Caucus, American Public Health Association Annual Meeting, Boston, Massachusetts.

Kennedy, E.L. & Davis, M.D. (1993), *Boots of Leather, Slippers of Gold: A History of the Lesbian Community,* New York, NY: Routledge, Inc.

Kessler, R.C., McGonagle, K.A., Zhao, S., Nelson, C.B., Hughes, M., Eshleman, S., Wittchen, H.U. & Kendler, K.S. (1994), Lifetime and 12-month prevalence of *DSM-III-R* psychiatric disorders in the U.S. *Archives General Psychiatry,* 51:8-19.

Kinsey, A., Pomeroy, W. & Martin, C. (1948), *Sexual Behavior in the Human Male.* Philadelphia, PA: Saunders.

Kinsey, A., Pomeroy, W., Martin, C. & Gebhard, P. (1953), *Sexual Behavior in the Human Female.* Philadelphia, PA: Saunders.

Krafft-Ebing, R. (1886), *Psychopathia Sexualis,* trans. H. Wedeck. New York: Putnam, 1965.

Krajeski, J. (1996), Homosexuality and the mental health professions. In: *Textbook of Homosexuality and Mental Health*, eds. R.P. Cabaj & T.S. Stein. Washington, DC: American Psychiatric Press, pp. 17-31.

Kruks, G. (1991), Gay and lesbian homeless/street youth: Special issues and concerns. *J. Adolescent Health*, 12:515-518.

Lawrence, A., Shaffer, J., Snow, W., Chase, C. & Headlam, B.T. (1996), Health care needs of transgender patients. *J. American Medical Association* 276:874.

Levy, E. (1992), Strengthening the coping resources of lesbian families. *Families in Society*, 73:23-31.

Liddle, B. (1996), Therapist sexual orientation, gender, and counseling practices as they relate to ratings of helpfulness by gay and lesbian consumers. *J. Counseling Psychology*, 43:394-401.

Marmor, J., ed. (1965), *Sexual Inversion: The Multiple Roots of Homosexuality*. New York: Basic Books.

McKirnan, D.J. & Peterson, P.L. (1989), Alcohol and drug use among homosexual men and women: Epidemiology and population characteristics. *Addictive Behaviors*, 14:545-553.

Meyer, I. (1995), Minority stress and mental health in gay men. *J. Health & Social Behavior*, 36:38-56.

Meyer, I.H. & Dean, L. (1995), Patterns of sexual behavior and risk-taking among young New York City gay men. *AIDS Education & Prevention*, 7:13-23.

Meyer, I.H. & Dean, L. (1998), Internalized homophobia, intimacy, and sexual behavior among gay and bisexual men. In: *Psychological Orientation: Understanding Prejudice Against Lesbians, Gay Men, and Bisexuals*, ed. G. Herek. Thousand Oaks, CA: Sage Publications.

National Association of State Mental Health Program Directors (2000), *Position Statement on Culturally Competent and Linguistically Appropriate Mental Health Services*. National Association of State Mental Health Program Directors Website (www.nasmhpd.org/linguist.htm.).

Oetjen, H. & Rothblum, E.D. (2000), When lesbians aren't gay: Factors affecting depression among lesbians. *J. Homosexuality*, 39:49-73.

Remafedi, G., Farrow, J.A. & Deischer, R.W. (1991), Risk factors for attempted suicide in gay and bisexual youth. *Pediatrics*, 87: 869-875.

Remafedi, G., French, S., Story, M., Resnick, M. & Blum, R. (1998), The relationship between suicide risk and sexual orientation: Results of a population-based study. *American J. Public Health*, 88(1):57-60.

Rich, G.L., Fowler, R.C., Young, D. & Blenkush, M. (1986), San Diego suicide study: Comparison of gay to straight males. *Suicide & Life-Threatening Behavior*, 16: 448-457.

Robins, L.E. & Regier, D.A. (1991), *Psychiatric Disorders in America: The Epidemiologic Catchment Area Study*. New York, NY: Free Press.

Rosario, V.A. (2003), An interview with Judd Marmor, MD. *J. Gay & Lesbian Psychotherapy*, 7(4):23-34.

Ross, M. (1990), The relationship between life events and mental health in homosexual men. *J. Clinical Psychology*, 46:402-411.

Rotheram-Borus, M., Hunter, J. & Rosario, M. (1994), Suicidal behavior and gay-related stress among gay and bisexual male adolescents. *J. Adolescent Research,* 9:498-508.

Sbordone, A.J. (2003), An interview with Charles Silverstein, PhD. *J. Gay & Lesbian Psychotherapy,* 7(4):49-61.

Scasta, D.L. (2002), John E. Fryer, MD, and the Dr. H. Anonymous episode. *J. Gay & Lesbian Psychotherapy,* 6(4):73-84.

Schneider, S.G., Farberow, N.L. & Kruks, G.N. (1989), Suicidal behavior in adolescent and young adult gay men. *Suicide & Life-Threatening Behavior,* 19:381-394.

Solarz, A.L., ed. (1999), *Lesbian Health: Current Assessment and Directions for the Future.* Washington, DC: Institute of Medicine, National Academy Press.

Sorensen L. & Roberts, S.J. (1997), Lesbian uses of and satisfaction with mental health services: Results from Boston Lesbian Health Project. *J. Homosexuality,* 33:35-49.

U.S. Department of Health and Human Services (DHHS) (1999), *Mental Health: A Report of the Surgeon General–Executive Summary.* Rockville, MD: DHHS, Center for Mental Health Services, Substance Abuse and Mental Health Services Administration, National Institutes of Health, National Institute of Mental Health.

U.S. Department of Health and Human Services (DHHS) (2000a), *Mental Health: Culture, Race, Ethnicity. Supplement to Mental Health: A Report of the Surgeon General–Executive Summary.* Rockville, MD: DHHS, Center for Mental Health Services, Substance Abuse and Mental Health Services Administration, National Institutes of Health, National Institute of Mental Health.

U.S. Department of Health and Human Services (DHHS) (2000a), *Healthy People 2010: Understanding and Improving Health. Second Edition.* Washington, DC: U.S. Government Printing Office.

Williams, J.B., Rabkin, J.G., Remien, R.H., Gorman, J.H & Ehrhardt, A.A. (1991), Multidisciplinary baseline assessment of homosexual men with and without human immunodeficiency virus infection: II. Standardized clinical assessment of current and lifetime psychopathology. *Archives General Psychiatry* 48:124-130.

Lesbian, Gay, Bisexual, and Transgender People Receiving Services in the Public Mental Health System: Raising Issues

Alicia Lucksted, PhD

SUMMARY. The growing literature about psychotherapy with LGBT clients rarely addresses serious mental illnesses or mental health care settings such as inpatient, psychosocial rehabilitation, day programs, or residential care. Nor does much of existing literature address the public mental health system. In 1997, the federal Center for Mental Health Services (part of Substance Abuse and Mental Health Services Administration and the federal Department of Health and Human Services) commissioned a review of current knowledge regarding the experiences, needs, and recommendations of LGBT people with serious mental illnesses. This article offers a summary of that multi-year project. Using qualitative methods and analysis, this study combines information from

Alicia Lucksted is affiliated with the Center for Mental Health Services Research, University of Maryland, 685 West Baltimore Street, MSTF Building, Room 300, Baltimore, MD 21201-1549 (E-mail: aluckste@psych.umaryland.edu).

Funding for this research project was provided by the Center for Mental Health Services, SAMHSA. The opinions expressed in this document reflect the personal opinions of the author and are not intended to represent the policies of the Center for Mental Health Services or other parts of the Federal Government. The author would like to thank Drs. Richard Goldberg and Diana Seybolt for their helpful suggestions regarding an earlier draft of this article.

[Haworth co-indexing entry note]: "Lesbian, Gay, Bisexual, and Transgender People Receiving Services in the Public Mental Health System: Raising Issues." Lucksted, Alicia. Co-published simultaneously in *Journal of Gay & Lesbian Psychotherapy* (The Haworth Medical Press, an imprint of The Haworth Press, Inc.) Vol. 8, No. 3/4, 2004, pp. 25-42; and: *Handbook of LGBT Issues in Community Mental Health* (ed: Ronald E. Hellman, and Jack Drescher) The Haworth Medical Press, an imprint of The Haworth Press, Inc., 2004, pp. 25-42. Single or multiple copies of this article are available for a fee from The Haworth Document Delivery Service [1-800-HAWORTH, 9:00 a.m. - 5:00 p.m. (EST). E-mail address: docdelivery@haworthpress.com].

25

archival sources, published and unpublished literature, and key informant interviews to highlight questions and themes important to the welfare of lesbian, gay, bisexual and transgender (LGBT) people receiving public/community mental health services. This paper raises issues about the experiences and needs of these populations that would benefit from further investigation, to help pique further inquiry, and to suggest constructive interim steps. *[Article copies available for a fee from The Haworth Document Delivery Service: 1-800-HAWORTH. E-mail address: <docdelivery@haworthpress.com> Website: <http://www.HaworthPress.com> © 2004 by The Haworth Press, Inc. All rights reserved.]*

KEYWORDS. Bisexual, gay, lesbian, mental health, mental health services, mental illness, public psychiatry, public sector, transgender

INTRODUCTION

There is a growing literature addressing psychotherapy with gay and lesbian clients, and bisexual and transgender clients to a lesser extent. This literature tends not to address the experiences of lesbian, gay, bisexual, or transgender (LGBT) people with serious mental illnesses[1] who require services and settings other than outpatient therapy (e.g., inpatient hospitalization, day or residential programs, psychosocial and vocational rehabilitation). Nor does much of the existing LGBT psychotherapy literature address the public mental health system. As part of an effort to set priorities regarding the diversity of people receiving mental health services for psychiatric disabilities, in 1997 the federal Center for Mental Health Services (part of Substance Abuse and Mental Health Services Administration and the federal Department of Health and Human Services) commissioned a review of current knowledge regarding the experiences and needs of LGBT people with serious mental illnesses. This article is a summary of that multi-year project.[2]

To date, published literature addressing these topics is extremely limited, despite repeated delineations of the need for such research. Hellman's (1996) essay in *Psychiatric Services* emphasized the need for attention to treatment issues for lesbians and gay men with serious mental illnesses. More than a decade earlier, Campbell and colleagues (1983) issued a similar call. More recently, Harris and Licata (2000) stressed these points and needs again. Cook (2000) more generally discusses the barriers to addressing sexuality in the context of psychiatric disabilities. However, Cabaj and Stein's *Textbook of Homosexuality and Mental Health* (1996) is virtually the only source on LGBT mental health that addresses the needs and experiences of LGBT people with serious mental illnesses in any depth. The only other readily available sources are Avery, Hellman and Sudderth's (2000) survey of 67 LGBT people receiving mental health services[3] and two earlier articles that describe group therapy interventions for LGBT people with serious mental illnesses in community mental health settings (Ball, 1994; Helfand, 1993).

This documentation and research lags behind other LGBT mental health topics for a number of reasons. LGBT people with serious mental illnesses are difficult to reach and to measure, given the multiple stigmas of psychiatric labels, LGBT identities, and the poverty common in the lives of people receiving services in the public system. Few resources have been available to mount substantial studies. Also, some researchers may be hesitant to study serious mental illness among LGBT people due to the history of LGBT identities being equated with psychopathology and fear of raising this specter again. The variables and issues involved are complex to operationalize: does one define "gay" based on self-identification, current or past sexual behavior, or participation in a sub-culture? Finally, what are the questions most in need of investigation?

While the text book essays and articles mentioned above are important beginnings, there is no coherent foundation of knowledge regarding LGBT people living with serious mental illnesses. The project summarized in this paper was designed to address one facet of this gap by specifying issues in need of inquiry, so as to help focus future work. Using qualitative methods of inquiry and analysis, the project combined the existing relevant professional literature with archival and unpublished sources, networking, and interview data from key informants (people with particular experience and knowledge on this topic). Consequently, this study cannot draw firm conclusions. Instead, its purposes are to help define the parameters of this topic area, to assist LGBT people receiving mental health services in having their voices heard, to spark professional interest, and suggest directions for research, service, and clinical inquiry and change.

METHODS

Data for this study came from various sources. The available professional, research and popular literatures relevant to the experiences and issues of LGBT clients of public mental health services were thoroughly reviewed. Sources from related areas of the academic and popular press were also considered, as was academic work on LGBT clients and psychotherapy.

Most information addressing the lives and needs of LGBT people with serious mental illnesses is found in local newsletters and periodicals, unpublished reports and essays, in-house materials, meeting proceedings, conference session recordings, personal correspondence, and more recently, web sites and email discussion groups. Therefore, in an effort to be as comprehensive and inclusive as possible, data for this study incorporated all of these sources. It also drew from conversations with many individuals and organizations: members of LGBT organizations, self-help advocacy and support organizations of people who consider themselves to have mental illnesses or psychiatric disabilities, people who have had extensive contact with the mental health system but do not identify as having a mental illness, activists, mental health service programs and clinicians of many types, professional organizations, related non-profit organizations, and government agencies. In all, more than 500 people and organizations were approached for their input, and more than half contributed suggestions, materials, and/or further contacts.

As part of this project, 35 key informants (Gilchrist, 1992) from across the U.S. were interviewed. Their perspectives included personal experiences as LGBT-identified users of various mental health services, advocates, community mental health workers, and professionals who provide services to LGBT people with serious mental illnesses. Their involvement was not an attempt to survey or randomly sample the relevant population as might be done in a quantitative study. Rather, the key informant method involves deliberately choosing "key" people who have extensive knowledge and experience in the area of interest, so that a project may be informed by the depth of their understanding. In this study, each key informant was recommended by other contacts as having specific, in-depth experiences and insights relevant to the project's focus. Each key informant was invited to take part, and then engaged in one or more open-ended conversations with the author about this project and their ideas, usually by telephone, but occasionally in person. Summary notes were taken during each conversation, including some verbatim quotations, and then mailed to the person for review. Once the key informant returned any comments and corrections, the revised notes became part of the study's data. Herein, key informants are cited as (KI *Name, Date of Interview*), using each person's choice of name, pseudonym, or "anonymous."

The ideas and information drawn from these published, unpublished, and first person sources make up the data for this project. These data were analyzed through conventional qualitative analysis methods of data reduction, emergent coding, and iterative integration (Miles and Huberman, 1994). That is, information from the disparate data sources were organized and integrated around the study's purpose through several steps. First, all materials were reviewed according to the study's guiding question: "What are the most important issues for LGBT people receiving services for serious mental illnesses, in the public system?" The "responses" embedded in each article, document, letter, or interview were then grouped into emergent categories forming a set of "codes" (Miles and Huberman, 1994) that also noted the interrelations among categories.

Once all data sources had contributed to the creation of this structured outline, its final version was applied to all the data. Passages, comments, and quotations across data sources were grouped together by code category (for example, "staff knowledge about LGBT issues") and then each category's overall meanings were distilled into a coherent summary of what the data had to "say" about that particular category of answer to the guiding question. Specific categories were then related to each other (e.g., B is a specific type of A) to further integrate the information into main themes. In qualitative research, staying true to the meanings expressed by one's data sources is considered crucial. Therefore, direct quotations are used whenever possible to present and illustrate the results. While all information was carefully examined and the resulting themes are robust, the data available for this study are incomplete and so conclusions must be considered tentative.

RESULTS

Given the project's rationale and methodology, its results are presented in the form of the major recurring themes and issues that emerged from analyzing and integrating the various information sources, accompanied by illustrative examples and quotations.

Addressing the Concerns of LGBT People with Serious Mental Illness: Diagnoses and Public Mental Health System Experience

Most sources noted that they find little to no recognition of LGBT issues in most public/community mental health settings. One said, "In the mental health system, we have to be closeted about being a sexual minority. There was no place we could feel at home, not be guarded because of fear of ridicule and rejection, and fully share who we are" (Holochuck, 1993. p. 17). Although this appears to be a dramatic statement, clients and clinicians alike from various locations and settings reported a belief that this was true. Prevalent opinion was that LGBT affirmative clinicians and programs often do not include people with serious mental illnesses within their scope of service or expertise, and that staff at many mental health programs do not know how to address the needs and dignity of LGBT people who come through their doors. Client-run mental health self-help and advocacy organizations were also described as often unknowledgeable and less than welcoming of the seriously mentally ill. In all cases, data suggest that efforts to fill in these knowledge gaps are rare, that staff and programs seldom have access to training on LGBT issues, and that clients' needs often go un-addressed.

Similarly, LGBT community organizations or "the gay community" are often experienced as paying little attention to the realities of LGBT people with serious psychiatric disabilities. Many diverse sources for this study described incidents in which LGBT community group members were unwelcoming to people in long-term mental health care, and widespread ignorance about mental illnesses.

Sources enthusiastically discussed people and groups they had found to be LGBT affirming on occasion, but repeatedly emphasized the overall dearth of attention to the issues, and the problems this creates. Many who work on behalf of LGBT people's welfare in the public mental health system echoed one key informant who said:

> *Any* knowledge you could put out through the report would help. There is a woeful lack of knowledge all over. Even places that are relatively gay friendly–even gay clinicians–don't know much about treating gay patients with serious mental illnesses. (KI Mary Barber, March 1998)

Addressing Sexuality in General

Another recurring theme in the data for this study was that mental health programs and facilities often seem to view *any* sexuality in a client's life as disturbed, or disturbing (e.g., Buckley and Hyde, 1997). Often, results suggest, sexuality is discussed only as a problem, such as warnings against unwanted pregnancy or HIV risk. There seems to be an underlying, often unspoken assumption that clients have, or should have, *no* sexuality (e.g., Trudel and Desjardins, 1992). For example, one key informant said:

> At the state hospital outpatient clinic, the staff tend to deny the sexuality of *all* patients. There's this sense of patients as children, who don't have a sexuality, or that it wouldn't be good for them to be sexual. Staff doesn't seem to want to deal with it. For example, a local community residence has a rule that residents cannot have sex in the house, [but] they don't really provide other guidelines or information, don't really address sexuality. It seems they just don't want to know about it–so, not in the house. (KI Mary Barer, March 1998)

Another key informant recalled:

> When I tried to develop a safe-sex workshop for clients, it took me *weeks* to get the staff to OK it. They were afraid that it would be too "stimulating" for the clients, would turn into a sex orgy. In reality, it is quite different. Clients are just *thankful* that someone is addressing sexuality issues in a positive open way–or at all. I've noticed the clients often really get organized and ask really good questions. (KI Orren Perlman, June 1998)

Moreover, lesbian, gay, and bisexual identities seem to be even more silenced and seen as problematic than heterosexual ones, especially given common misconceptions about LGBT people.

Staff Knowledge and Attitudes

A third prevailing theme that emerged from this study's data was the perceived high level of anti-LGBT stereotypes and ignorance among staff and programs in community mental health systems. Key informants and other sources spoke in appreciation of mental health workers of all disciplines who are familiar with and affirming of LGBT identities. They lauded programs that have institutionalized affirming practices, but noted that they are very rare. Instead, it was reported to be common that mental health programs seem to assume that LGBT clients do not exist, that all clients are tacitly assumed to be heterosexual. One person described this:

> Even most progressive CMH programs, at least here, don't take into consideration that you may be a sexual minority. Especially day treatment programs and housing programs. A number of clients have experienced it–in day programs, outpatient clinics, inpatient units, community residences, boarding homes–sexual orientation is just never taken into account. (KI Audrey Grifel, March 1998)

A related theme was that of experiences with mental health workers who give the distinct impression that they do not understand, do not like, and do not want to deal with LGBT people. While not addressing attitudes towards LGBT people with serious mental illnesses in particular, published commentary (e.g., Forstein, 1993; Saunders, et al., 2001) and research regarding the attitudes of mental health and social service workers towards LGBT people suggests high levels of anti-LGBT misconceptions and aversion, accompanied by gradual improvements over time (Smith, 1993; Berkman and Zinberg, 1997; Hayes and Erkis, 2000). In this study, data sources reported that it is common for LGBT mental health clients to encounter assumptions that LGBT people are either HIV positive, sexual predators, man-hating, swishy, butch, confused, sick, or other such stereotypes. These experiences were mentioned again and again in written first person accounts and interviews. Two examples:

> Some [staff] see something bad in the gay community and (1) stereotype us by assuming that we're all like that just because we're gay. Then (2) they don't even *think* about how many really bad problems are going on that impact the gay community and cause the things they're seeing–

how homophobia, AIDS, problems with families, isolation, all that, effect people. (KI Angel Olmeda, July, 1998)

It took me a long time to build my life back up again after that [a disastrous phone call to family made at the insistence of her social worker]. I believe that the social worker did not really have any idea about the issues of a family totally disowning someone for being gay–how strong homophobia is, and that it is not going to be "cured" by a phone call. (KI Lynne D'Orsay, February, 1998)

One published commentary emphasized that such experiences are detrimental to the clients' care and health:

For individuals diagnosed with serious mental illness who are LGBT, homophobic attitudes among providers of mental health services, and mental health programs which are heterosexist, create barriers to recovery and detract from the effectiveness of treatment and support services. (Chassman, 1996, p. 1-2)

Key informants also raised the issue of mental health workers who exhibit a superficial semblance of sensitivity, but shy away or even pathologize clients' attempts to discuss LGBT issues outside the clinician's limited "comfort zone." As one person summarized it:

Mental health workers often put on how advanced, knowledgeable, OK they are with LGBT and HIV topics. But if you scratch the surface at all, you find they don't know much, they really aren't comfortable with it, and they don't want to deal with it–with others' issues or their own. They're just trying to appear sensitive without really being so. (KI Bill Adams, July 1998)

Others described experiences with therapists and other staff who tended to assume or insist that being LGBT is "no big deal," regardless of what the client presents, or that it is the focal clinical problem even when the client says it is not. The data for this study even more robustly emphasize that many people working in mental health systems (including some who are gay or lesbian) are still especially uninformed about bisexual and transgender people, making it especially difficult for members of these groups to find good mental health care. As one concrete illustration:

As I was going along, most often my therapists didn't know anything about being transgender. I had to educate them. It really bothered me, and changed the whole therapy dynamic and takes away from the trust you feel, and the time spent on *you*, even though that's why you are there. (KI Melanie Spritz, June 1998)

Peer Intolerance

Key informants and other data sources said that harassment and belittlement of people known to be lesbian, gay, bisexual and/or transgender by other clients is common. Diverse sources reported experiencing and/or observing the same pattern across many different mental health settings: While a few clients are positive and many are neutral toward LGBT peers, verbal derogation from those who are uncomfortable or hostile towards LGBT people is abundant, threats are not infrequent, and staff often seem to passively excuse both. One person commented,

> Patients in the system also panic; there is *lots* of homophobia and transphobia, and attacks and harassment. And the staff will usually ignore it, condone it by their inactivity. (KI Anonymous D., May 1998)

There were scattered accounts of staff harassment as well. Varied sources also reported that when LGBT individuals with mental illnesses go to local self-help organizations or LGBT community groups for peer support, they often encounter disregard or discrimination there as well. An important sub-theme was that misconceptions about HIV may be an important component of peer hostility towards LGBT people. For example, Anonymous W. said:

> In any kind of group situation [being LGBT] is still somewhat of an anathema–there are still repercussions of being forthright, especially since the HIV health crisis. That's one assumption made about people in a psych hospital–that everyone is HIV positive. And, therefore, patients will go out of the way to avoid being associated with anyone, any identity that is associated with HIV–like gay men. (KI, May 1998)

Family Stress and Safety Net

People with serious mental illnesses must often rely on family members for help with housing, finances, and emotional support, either as a matter of course or as a back up "last resort" (Schene, van Wijngaarden, and Koeter, 1998). However, information gathered in this study suggests that some LGBT people receiving mental health care may not be able to count on this "safety net" due to familial conflict or rejection regarding their sexual orientation or gender identity. As one woman explained:

> I, for example, came out to my family 13 years ago and was immediately disowned. Despite efforts to contact them, cards and gifts sent, etc., I have never seen another single member of my family again, even though my sister, nieces and mother live only 35 miles away. I was told that I would be arrested for trespassing if I tried to visit them. Although extreme, this is not entirely atypical of the [LGBT] consumers' experience. (KI Lynne D'Orsay, February 1998)

Others may have access to their families, but at a high price of stress and isolation:

> I am bisexual and living with an abusive father (finances keep me at home). I cannot, at least for now, even hint of such a possibility to my immediate family. There's been enough trouble. I fear they would call me crazy, just for [being bisexual]. (Haller, 1996, p. 1)

Continued Pathologization of LGBT Identities

Although "homosexuality" was removed from the *Diagnostic and Statistical Manual* of psychiatric disorders in 1973, the data in this study suggests that the pathologizing of non-heterosexual identities still lingers. Various data sources report encountering mental health professionals who consider LGBT identities to be illnesses, delusions–or some other psychiatric symptom–or a level of arrested psychosocial development. One advocate emphasized that "The fundamental issue is *still* that it is *not* a pathology, and the mental health system still is not as accepting as it ought to be of this" (KI Anonymous W., May 1998).

Several specific points emerged under this broad theme of continued pathologization. First, the results of this study suggest that a heterosexual standard of mental health may be affecting the care of LGBT patients. There were many comments and examples of heterosexuality being considered healthier than lesbian, gay, or bisexual orientations, and of LGBT individuals having their overall mental health evaluated in part by how "straight" and "gender appropriate" they seemed to the clinicians. For example:

> When I was at _____ Hospital, I got in a lot of trouble and was considered seriously depressed because I refused to put on make-up or act in other ways they considered appropriate for [heterosexual] females. I was openly gay at the time. (KI Anonymous P., September 1998)

> While in hospital in _____, staff said they'd take it as a good sign that I was ready for discharge only when I was willing to see a psychiatrist they chose and stop seeing the gay therapist I had chosen. (Michael Deacon in Deacon, Rea, Largey, 1991)

Second, the data frequently included reports of unfamiliarity and stereotypes leading some mental health clinicians to interpret adaptive or neutral behaviors by LGBT clients as pathological. For example, reasonable self-protectiveness or anxiety about encountering homophobia was mis-interpreted as clinical paranoia; bisexual identity was interpreted per se as an indicator of personality disorder (KI Orren Perlman, June, 1998). Key informant Steve Hartman (May 1998) reported observing that the style of self expression adopted by some gay men called "acting like a queen," which is seen by LGBT people as a way of coping with stress, expressing frustration, or being humorous, is sometimes pathologized as "histrionic" and a symptom of borderline personality disorder.

Third, several experienced clinicians noted that older LGBT patients sometimes have difficulty accessing needed care due to past hurtful experiences. For example:

> It is especially poignant with older clients who have experienced lots of abuse in the mental health system in decades past. They are very wary about the Mental Health system–period, and about being out certainly. Usually they are not out at all on the unit, and are reluctant to talk about it openly. I think this is due to years of misuse at the hands of the mental health system. In our LGBT support group, elderly gay and lesbian clients have talked about receiving ECT and aversion therapy electric shocks applied to their genitalia when they respond to same sex erotica. Those with chronic mental illnesses like schizophrenia, for example, talk about not being seen as cured or the exacerbation being seen as in remission because the client "still" maintained an attraction to members of their own sex. (KI Orren Perlman, June 1998)

Information Regarding LGBT Community Resources

During this project, a wide range of data sources raised concerns that mental health programs often have no knowledge of LGBT-affirmative community resources in their locale and frequently ignore LGBT issues when crafting treatment and discharge plans. For example, one gay man told of asking whether the day program he was being referred to was welcoming of LGBT people, or if he would need to plan to protect himself from potential hostility-issues which had not occurred to the referring staff. Similarly, a transgender person reported asking whether a given group home was safe for transgender people, and a bisexual woman asked for help finding a bisexual-affirmative outpatient therapist or support group. In each instance, staff could not answer the question or request, and sometimes reacted defensively when asked. One staff person recalled, "when I and another staff-person did a [staff] in-service on GLB issues, people asked very basic questions and did not know of even the most common community resources we listed" (KI Mary Barber, May 1998). A peer advocate concurred, "I've worked with clients who felt there was no awareness and acknowledgement by staff that sexual orientation is an important part of their [clients'] lives and would/should be an integral part of their recovery and treatment" (KI Audrey Grifel, March 1998).

Inpatient and Residential Services

Recurring anecdotes suggest that residential mental health settings may be among the most problematic for LGBT people with mental illnesses due to close quarters, lack of privacy, and around-the-clock proximity among residents. Sources in various locations repeatedly described being treated with suspicion, assumed to be a sexual predator toward same-gender staff and patients (particularly roommates), and constantly scrutinized. A wide range of sources noted that there is considerable harassment, discrimination, and even physical assault of LGBT residents in some inpatient and residential settings. Several examples illustrate this issue:

> Within any residential system–psychiatric, shelters, domestic violence shelters–it is gender binary: women, men. Which dorm? Which wing? Which bathroom? If you don't fit easily, the staff get very upset. Other clients too. And it's very, very frightening for the transgender client–the level of alienation and hostility, and danger, they can be in. (KI Anonymous A, June 1998)

> One person related a time when he felt attracted to another man who slept nearby on the hospital ward. He asked the nurses if he could sleep in another area, and had to tell them the reason. He was given another place to sleep, but the next day everyone on the floor knew about the request. In fact, the story had grown as it was passed around so that some people thought he had been "caught" in an intimate act with the man or had aggressively pursued him. He recalled that a doctor said to him, "scum like you should be locked up," and was not interested in hearing his version of the events. (A. Lucksted, field notes from group discussion, May, 1998)

> Just recently in our [self-help] group a 23-year-old Latina woman in chronic treatment, in a residential program, was outed by a person she thought was a friend, and who she had told she was a lesbian in confidence. The friend went to the whole house, and the woman was harassed a lot and was very upset. We spent most of the afternoon meeting of our group helping support her. (KI Bert Coffman, May 1998)

In addition, many data sources alleged that inpatient/residential staff often look the other way or blame the victim when discrimination occurs. Others told of staff participating in harassment or in creating a hostile environment. For example, several related stories of staff either forbidding clients from disclosing their LGBT identity to anyone in the residence on pain of expulsion or forcing a new resident to disclose his/her identity to everyone, regardless of privacy, clinical, or safety concerns (KI Zappalorti Society Meeting, August 1998). Others told of staff not considering a same-gender relationship legitimate "family."

LGBT-Affirmative Services

In addition to lauding individual mental health workers who are well informed and experienced in providing care to LGBT people with serious mental illnesses, data sources for this study also praised and expressed thanks for mental health settings that bring LGBT-affirming qualities to a programmatic level. Key informants and written first-person accounts consistently emphasized that when a mental health program is knowledgeable about, comfortable with, and sensitive to LGBT clients' needs, clients feel safer and more at ease, thereby facilitating trust in therapeutic relationships, engagement in treatment, and openness on the client's part. They also stressed that in LGBT-affirmative environments, LGBT identities become less of an issue in treatment, because LGBT clients do not have to be constantly vigilant around identity, self-presentation issues, or the potential for adverse reactions from others. This allows them to better concentrate on the mental health needs they are there to address (see also Burling, 2002). In addition, they argue, services in such settings better address the clients' real-life needs and priorities, and are more tailored to that individual. For example, one person described his reactions to attending an LGBT-affirming program:

> Here people are more comfortable with each other, more knowledgeable about themselves and issues, more aware of social problems, and more involved with each other. They don't take just a medical view [of] "medicate and go." So, I feel I can be more up-front regarding all the complex parts of homosexuality, and of HIV. Communication is more open, so that if there is some tension or problem it can be put on the table; communication is much less defensive. (KI Angel Olmeda, July 1998)

Several mental health professionals offered other positive benefits of openness:

> Instead of pretending [sexual activity on the unit, despite official prohibitions] doesn't happen, [our unit] tries to address it openly. We encour-

age people to think about, talk about, and express sexual feelings in thoughtful, adult ways. (KI Steve Hartman, May 1998)

Posting information, posters, books, brochures on LGBT issues and organizations is part of our creating an affirmative environment. (KI Ron Hellman, June 1998)

There needs to be a way to make sure we have clinicians who can provide the services that are needed, including gay-affirmative MH services. It's not the sexual orientation of the trainees that matters, but their willingness to learn the information, and their interest in being educated and sensitive in this area. (KI Anonymous P., September 1998)

Finally, there has been a slowly developing movement among LGBT mental health care recipients to speak up and organize locally, and sometimes nationally, to support each other and advocate for more inclusive and LGBT-positive mental health services and self-help groups (Rogers, 2002). Individuals and several small organizations such as the Zappalorti Society in Manhattan (KI Bert Coffman, May 1998), Hearts & Ears, Inc. in Baltimore (Hearts & Ears, Inc., 2002), and the Pink and Black Triangle Society (Project Return, 2001) are working to provide LGBT-affirming "spaces" within the current mental health system and self-help movements, while also working to improve both.

DISCUSSION

People receiving mental health services in inpatient, psychosocial rehabilitation, and similar settings are usually there because they need assistance beyond what is available through natural supports or outpatient psychotherapy. Further, many receiving services through the public health system have few other resources. Therefore, we might be especially concerned for their welfare and about the impact of poor treatment or discrimination based on sexual orientation, gender identity, or other sources (Cabaj, 1995; Cabaj and Stein, 1996). Although this study does not document the prevalence or breadth of these problems, by consulting a wide variety of information sources and experienced people and organizations, it raises recurring issues and questions that deserve further examination.

Significantly, it raises concern that the needs and welfare of LGBT people with serious mental illnesses are being neglected in our current public/community mental health service systems. For example, while prevalent standards of care call for helping clients create a meaningful adult life that is integrated into their community, many mental health settings seem ambivalent and uncomfortable addressing sexuality in the lives of their clients. Sexuality may be discussed in terms of avoiding exploitation, pregnancy or STDs, but rarely is this balanced by programming to help clients create sustaining, adult intimate relationships. There does not appear to be any training for staff in these topics. Consequently, if positive views of heterosexuality are de facto taboo, lesbian, gay, and bisexual orientations and transgender identities seem to be even more so.

Similarly, standards of community-embedded care call for discharge and "integration" plans that help clients connect with facets of the local community that are important to them, such as employment, religious centers, cultural organizations, and recreation opportunities. Yet, data sources for this study held strong opinions that connecting to LGBT community organizations or finding an LGBT-welcoming place of worship is rarely–if ever, included in an LGBT client's care plan. In other words, mental health programs seldom think of LGBT organizations as valuable parts of the wider community for themselves or their clients.

Coping with oppression is taxing, regardless of one's setting or resources (for examples, see Bell and Nkomo, 1998; Dunbar, 2001; Karlsen and Nazroo, 2002). For LGBT people confronting serious mental health challenges, disregard or discrimination in the mental health system can be unsettling in settings that are supposed to be places of help and healing. Various individual LGBT mental health clients and observers who contributed to this study said that facing LGBT-insensitive environments requires expending tremendous energy to manage one's identity and self-presentation. Significant effort is required to manage fear, anxiety, and the unhelpful reactions of people from whom one might hope to get support: program staff, peers, and family.

It is not implausible to assume that such stresses can distract a client's energy and attention from recovering his or her mental health, preclude bringing one's "whole self" into treatment, and may also lead to frustration, anger, isolation, and depression (as found with other experiences of discrimination). The current study raises particular concern about inpatient and residential programs in this regard. Anti-LGBT biases may also create barriers to needed services, either because services for LGBT individuals cannot be found, or because an individual is reluctant to enter into a program or system that s/he knows or suspects to be hostile. These assumptions are based on anecdotal information, and, while plausible, must necessarily await confirmation through further evaluation and research.

Finally, LGBT issues do not only affect LGBT people. Being perceived as fitting a stereotype can be enough to lead others to presume one is gay, regardless of one's actual sexual identity. Key informant Bill Adams (July 1998) said, "Shelters cannot deal with men who are at all effeminate–they get beaten up" regardless of their sexual orientation or gender identity.

We do not yet know the extent or contours of many of the problems and issues raised in this study, nor do we know much about what LGBT-affirming services for people with serious mental illnesses would look like, what would be needed to bring about changes, and what effects they would have. Efforts to draw together a base of knowledge that would foster programs of research and other avenues of inquiry to answer these questions need to be supported and disseminated widely.

However, waiting for extensive confirmation also seems unwise given the many troubling experiences conveyed here and elsewhere, as well as the stories told of LGBT-affirming experiences. There are numerous constructive steps that can be taken in the meantime: As we work to develop a knowledge base, asking questions of our local mental health programs and self-help/advocacy groups can raise consciousness and clarify local needs. Adapting the well-developed body of research regarding LGBT-affirming psychotherapy to other settings can lend weight and direction to our efforts. Working to make LGBT resources more available to programs, staff, and clients alike and educating our LGBT communities about the detriments of stigma regarding mental illness, can begin to address needs in locally relevant ways.[4] Carried out in a thoughtful iterative fashion, such efforts can address immediate needs, while also providing important input to our wider research and systems inquiry, which can then refine our clinical and systems-change efforts.

NOTES

1. "Serious mental illness," "serious and persistent mental Illness," "psychiatric disabilities" and related terms refer to mental/emotional disturbances, usually involving DSM-IV Axis I diagnoses, that substantially impair a person's daily functioning and enacting of usual adult roles, and in which this impairment persists or frequently recurs over long periods of time (years).

2. The full report (~100pgs) is available from the author at 410/706-2490 or *aluckste@psych.umaryland.edu.*

3. It indicated that respondents would benefit from services more tailored to their needs.

4. One example of a local workshop being offered free to psychosocial programs may be requested from the author.

REFERENCES

Avery, A.M., Hellman, R.E. & Sudderth, L.K. (2001), Satisfaction with mental health services among sexual minorities with major mental illness. *American J. Public Health*, 91(6):990-991.

Ball, S. (1994), A group model for gay and lesbian clients with chronic mental illness. *Social Work*, 39(1):109-115.

Bell, E.L.J.E. & Nkomo, S.M. (1998), Armoring: Learning to withstand racial oppression. *J. Comparative Family Studies*, 29(2):285-292.

Berkman, C.S. & Zinberg, G. (1997), Homophobia and heterosexism in social workers. *Social Work*, 42(2):319-322.

Buckley, P.F. & Hyde, J.L. (1997), State hospitals' responses to the sexual behavior of psychiatric inpatients. *Psychiatric Services*, 48(3):398-399.

Burling, S. (2002, Sept. 15), Special wards lend aid to mentally ill gays. *Philadelphia Inquirer*, p. A1.

Cabaj, R.P. (1995), Sexual orientation and the addictions. *J. Gay & Lesbian Psychotherapy*, 2(3):97-117.

Cabaj, R.P. & Stein, T.S. (1996), *Textbook of Homosexuality and Mental Health*. Washington, DC: American Psychiatric Press.

Campbell, H.D., Hinkle, D.O., Sandlin, P. & Moffic, H.S. (1983), A sexual minority: Homosexuality and mental health care. *American J. Social Psychiatry*, 3(2): 26-35.

Chassman, J. (1996), Deviance or diversity. *The Gay & Lesbian "Consumer" Newsletter*, 1(2):1-2.

Cook, J.A. (2000), Sexuality and people with psychiatric disabilities, *Sexuality & Disability*, 18(3):195-206.

Deacon, M., Rea, I. & Largey, M. (1991), Psychiatric survivors: Surviving bigotry [panel discussion recorded from community cable access TV]. Copies available from MC Video Productions, P.O. Box 3012, Madison, WI 53704-0012.

Dunbar, E. (2001), Counseling practices to ameliorate the effects of discrimination and hate events: Toward a systematic approach to assessment and intervention. *Counseling Psychologist*, 29 (2):279-307.

Forstein, M. (1993), President's column. *Association of Gay & Lesbian Psychiatrists Newsletter*, 18(4):3.

Gilchrist, V.J. (1992), Key informant interviews. In: *Doing Qualitative Research: Research Methods for Primary Care, Vol. 3*, eds. B.F. Crabtree & W.L. Miller. Thousand Oaks, CA: Sage Publications, Inc., pp. 70-89.

Haller, J. (1996), Coming out–sideways. *The Gay & Lesbian "Consumer" Newsletter*, 1(4):1.

Harris, H.L. & Licata, F. (2000), From fragmentation to integration: Affirming the identities of culturally diverse, mentally ill lesbians and gay men. *J. Gay & Lesbian Social Services: Issues in Practice, Policy & Research*, 11(4):93-103.

Hayes, J.A. & Erkis, A.J. (2000), Therapist homophobia, client sexual orientation, and source of client HIV infection as predictors of therapist reactions to clients with HIV. *J. Counseling Psychology*, 47(1):71-78.

Hearts & Ears, Inc. (2002), A letter to friends and members. *Hearts & Ears Newsletter*, 3(1):1,6, June [Newsletter and information available from Hearts & Ears, Inc. at www.heartsandears.org or tel: 410/837-7778].

Helfand, K.L. (1993), Therapeutic considerations in structuring a support group for the mentally ill gay and lesbian population. *J. Gay & Lesbian Psychotherapy*, 2(1): 65-76.

Hellman, R.E. (1996), Issues in the treatment of lesbian women and gay men with chronic mental illnesses. *Psychiatric Services*, 47(10):1093-1098.

Holochuck, S. (1993), Mad, queer and proud!: Psychiatric survivor and activist Steven Holochuck speaks out. *The Lavender Network*, 90:15-17.

Karlsen, S. & Nazroo, J.Y. (2002), Agency and structure: The impact of ethnic identity and racism on the health of ethnic minority people. *Sociology of Health and Illness*, 24(1):1-20.

Miles, M.H. & Huberman, A.M. (1994), *Qualitative Data Analysis: An Expanded Sourcebook*. Thousand Oaks, CA: Sage Publications.

Project Return, (2001), *Pink and Black Triangle Society for Gays and Lesbians with Psychiatric Disability*, Unpublished pamphlet, available from Project Return, 1138 Wilshire Blvd, Suite 100, Los Angeles, CA 90017-1705, 323/413-1130, prtns@aol.com.

Rogers, S. (2002), Growth of LGBT consumer/survivor movement slow but sure. *The Key: National Mental Health Consumers' Self-Help Clearinghouse Newsletter*, 7(2):4-6.

Saunders, D., Bewley, S., Bolton, J., Playdon, Z.J., Oxley, J., von Fragstein, M. & Harris, R. (2001), Commentary: The medical profession should face up to its own homophobia. *British Medical Journal*, 322(7283): 424-425.

Schene, A.H., van Wijngaarden, B. & Koeter, M.W.J. (1998), Family caregiving in schizophrenia: Domains and distress. *Schizophrenia Bulletin*, 24: 609-618.

Smith, G.B. (1993), Homophobia and attitudes towards gay men and lesbians by psychiatric nurses. *Archives Psychiatric Nursing*, 7(6):377-384.

Trudel, G. & Desjardins, G. (1992). Staff reactions toward the sexual behaviors of people living in institutional settings. *Sexuality & Disability*, 10(3):173-188.

Advocating for Health and Human Services: The New York Experience

Sheila A. Healy, MPA

SUMMARY. This article describes how the Empire State Pride Agenda Foundation, working in partnership with the New York State LGBT Health and Human Services Network, developed and utilized education, advocacy and community organizing strategies to overcome the barriers of political and cultural opposition, inadequate knowledge about the health care needs of the community, and heterocentric models of health care to secure governmental recognition of the health and wellness needs of the lesbian, gay, bisexual and transgender (LGBT) community in the form of targeted funding for LGBT health and human service needs. This partnership created an effective vehicle for state recognition of non-HIV LGBT service needs. In five years, this partnership has generated a total of $10.7 million in state funding for a wide range of services including primary and preventive health as well as mental health care, crime victim assistance, counseling and support services to LGBT people across the state including youth, seniors, people of color and transgender individuals. It should be stressed, however, that the health

Sheila A. Healy was the Program Director of the Empire State Pride Agenda Foundation, the non-partisan education, research, and advocacy arm of ESPA. She is presently the Executive Director of the National Association of Lesbian, Gay, Bisexual and Transgender Community Centers in Washington, DC.

Address correspondence to: Sheila A. Healy, 1325 Massachusetts Avenue NW, Suite 600, Washington, DC 20005 (E-mail: NALGBTCC@hotmail.com).

[Haworth co-indexing entry note]: "Advocating for Health and Human Services: The New York Experience." Healy, Sheila A. Co-published simultaneously in *Journal of Gay & Lesbian Psychotherapy* (The Haworth Medical Press, an imprint of The Haworth Press, Inc.) Vol. 8, No. 3/4, 2004, pp. 43-66; and: *Handbook of LGBT Issues in Community Mental Health* (ed: Ronald E. Hellman, and Jack Drescher) The Haworth Medical Press, an imprint of The Haworth Press, Inc., 2004, pp. 43-66. Single or multiple copies of this article are available for a fee from The Haworth Document Delivery Service [1-800-HAWORTH, 9:00 a.m. - 5:00 p.m. (EST). E-mail address: docdelivery@haworthpress.com].

http://www.haworthpress.com/web/JGLP
Digital Object Identifer: 10.1300/J236v08n03_04

and human service needs of the LGBT community far exceed the total amount of funding provided by New York State. *[Article copies available for a fee from The Haworth Document Delivery Service: 1-800-HAWORTH. E-mail address: <docdelivery@haworthpress.com> Website: <http://www.HaworthPress.com>* © *2004 by The Haworth Press, Inc. All rights reserved.]*

KEYWORDS. Advocacy, agencies, agenda, bisexual, budget, education, Empire State Pride Foundation, foundation, gay, government, health, human services, legislature, lesbian, mental health, network, New York State, state, transgender

INTRODUCTION

In discrete ways, New York State has funded the health and wellness needs of the lesbian and gay community for over two decades. However, official state recognition of these needs has been a relatively recent phenomenon. [1]

This article describes how the Empire State Pride Agenda Foundation, working in partnership with the New York State Lesbian, Gay, Bisexual and Transgender Health and Human Services Network, developed and utilized education, advocacy and community organizing strategies to overcome the barriers of political and cultural opposition, inadequate knowledge about the health care needs of the community, and heterocentric models of health care to secure governmental recognition of the health and wellness needs of the lesbian, gay, bisexual and transgender (LGBT) community in the form of targeted funding for LGBT health and human service needs. [2]

NEW YORK STATE FUNDING HISTORY

The first time that New York State provided any type of funding for the lesbian and gay community was in the early 1980s to support HIV education, counseling and prevention. This funding came as a direct result of efforts made by advocates to get state officials to respond to the impact of the AIDS epidemic on the community. However, it was not until 1994 that New York State included an appropriation in the state budget expressly targeting lesbian and gay men for HIV/AIDS education programs, as well as alcohol and drug abuse prevention. This funding was largely a product of the efforts made by a handful of relatively new but politically sophisticated New York City-based lesbian and gay organizations to advocate for more public recognition of the community's AIDS crisis.

At the same time, New York State had begun to provide a fairly limited number of lesbian and gay specific grassroots, community-based organizations with funding for non-HIV/AIDS-related services through state agencies such as the Office of Children and Family Services (the former Division for Youth), the Office of Alcoholism and Substance Abuse Services, the Division of Criminal Justice Services and the Crime Victims Board.

Another fifteen years passed before New York State officially recognized that lesbian and gay health and social service needs extended beyond HIV/AIDS. It was around that time that the State Department of Health issued a Request for Proposals for the Lesbian and Gay Health and Human Services Initiative. This initiative was made possible by one-time discretionary funding of $1 million provided by Governor George Pataki for non-HIV related programs that promoted "wellness and access to health and human services for lesbian and gay individuals and their families."[3]

This first public step towards governmental recognition of the community's non-HIV needs resulted from community members' acknowledgment of the need to become better organized to achieve their advocacy goals. In the process, they essentially pioneered a new advocacy strategy that had not yet been replicated in any other state. The strategy consisted of creating a statewide network of lesbian and gay service providers. This network then established a partnership with New York's statewide political advocacy organization, the Empire State Pride Agenda (the "Pride Agenda").

This partnership, still unique in the nation, is operated under the aegis of the Empire State Pride Agenda Foundation (the "Foundation," see below). It created a vehicle for pursuing state recognition of non-HIV LGBT service needs. In just over four years, the annual level of funding grew from $1 million to $3.7 million, or $10.7 million in cumulative state funding for a wide range of non-HIV-related health and human services.

This relationship stands apart because it utilizes the expertise of both social service providers and those with political expertise to access the resources of government. The relationship is the result of a recognition by service providers that simply expressing a need for assistance does not result in a response by government, and a recognition by governmental advocates that service providers can humanize needs in a compelling way.

BUILDING THE INSTITUTIONAL CAPACITY FOR ADVOCACY

The Network

The New York City Lesbian and Gay Community Services Center (later renamed the LGBT Community Center) and the Hetrick-Martin Institute were instrumental in establishing the first statewide coalition of lesbian and gay human service providers in New York over a decade ago. Known today as the New York State Lesbian, Gay, Bisexual and Transgender Health and Human

Services Network (the "Network"–see Appendix), the coalition was created in response to concerns about funding cuts that were then threatening lesbian and gay community-based organizations. At the time, the community recognized that while it was able to increase or protect HIV-specific programs, it was not as successful in obtaining funding for non-HIV programs. The Network was charged with the task of addressing: (a) the reality that government had failed to meet the pressing and unmet needs of New York State's large LGBT community; and, (b) the need for the community to organize and insure that state government begin to target the LGBT community for funding of non-HIV/AIDS health and social services.

The Foundation

The Foundation was established in late 1995 as the non-partisan research, education and advocacy arm of the Pride Agenda to support and enhance the efforts of LGBT communities throughout New York State and to advocate for their political goals and health and human service needs. Recognizing the importance of the Network in achieving its mission, the Foundation incorporated the Network in-house as its first major program in the same year that it was founded.

The Foundation administers and funds the Network as an independent coalition of 50 diverse health and social service providers that offer a wide array of community-based services to LGBT individuals across the state. These services include primary, preventive and mental health care, crime victim assistance, crisis intervention and family counseling, social support, and education. These organizations serve upstate and downstate populations, urban and rural, and specific subpopulations within the LGBT community, including youth, seniors, people of color, and transgender individuals. Embedded in the mission and goals of the Foundation is the recognition that building and strengthening an effective statewide network of grassroots LGBT organizations is a key to ameliorating the long-standing health and social welfare challenges facing the LGBT community, and to overcoming the barriers to quality health and social services for LGBT people and their families.

STRATEGIES AND TACTICS

State of the State Reports

The Foundation, in collaboration with the Network, published its first annual State of the State report in 1999. The purpose of this report was to increase awareness among New York's elected and appointed officials of the concerns and struggles of LGBT New Yorkers and their families, and to educate them about the most pressing health, mental health and human service needs of the LGBT community.

The report represented the first time that the LGBT community had submitted a public policy document to New York State that described the non-HIV social, economic and health-related challenges created by many years of discrimination against the community. It documented the inadequacy of the existing services delivered to the LGBT community by mainstream providers through denial of care, poor or inappropriate care, and lack of providers trained in the unique health and social service concerns of LGBT people.

As the first formal document focused at the state level to link the community's mental health problems to bias and discrimination, it stated:

> Mental health needs can be heightened by estrangement from families, stress, the effects of hostility, violence, or anti-gay abuse, the toll of homophobia on self-esteem, and the lack of social support for gay family structures. Studies have found heightened rates of depression among gay men, possibly linked to the emotional burdens of HIV/AIDS, and several studies have indicated that lesbian and gay adults, youth, and elders are at increased risk for suicide.[4]

Also designed to educate New York State legislators and policy makers, the 2000 State of the State report included documentation from a wide range of sources on the pervasive impact of anti-gay discrimination on the LGBT community's health and wellness in nine functional areas: health, mental health, substance abuse and alcoholism, bias violence, domestic violence, education, youth, seniors and social services. In this capacity, it stated:

> Lacking legal protection, and economically vulnerable, LGBT New Yorkers live in an atmosphere of isolation, hostility, and anti-gay stigma and violence. Our health care issues are compounded by this anti-gay discrimination. Discrimination by providers, inadequate services, lack of access to family health insurance coverage, and fear of repercussion from homophobic social service institutions make LGBT New Yorkers less likely to seek care. They are also less likely to receive appropriate care when they do seek it out. As a direct result of societal stigma and inadequate care, LGBT people are at increased risk for a host of health care problems.[5]

The 2001 State of the State report profiled ten Network organizations that had been awarded grants under the 1998 Lesbian and Gay Health and Human Services Initiative, and highlighted steps taken for the first time by state agencies to improve the lives and well-being of LGBT New Yorkers in response to the advocacy work of the Foundation and the Network. The report noted:

At the same time, state agencies have begun to realize that in order to truly fulfill their mission of promoting the well-being of all of New York's citizens, they must improve their delivery of services to those citizens who are lesbian, gay, bisexual and transgender. Collaboration between these agencies and members of the LGBT community has produced remarkable results. Sensitivity trainings have been implemented; requests for proposals have targeted gay youth; lesbian and gay service providers have been consulted on planning documents. Much more remains to be done.[6]

GOVERNMENTAL ADVOCACY IN THE EXECUTIVE BRANCH

The Foundation/Network partnership has focused its primary advocacy efforts on eight agencies within the Executive Branch of New York State government that are responsible for meeting New Yorkers health and human service needs: the State Office for the Aging, the Office of Alcoholism and Substance Abuse Services, the Office for the Prevention of Domestic Violence, the State Education Department, the Office of Mental Health, the Department of Health, the Division of Criminal Justice Services and the Office of Children and Family Services.

The goal of the advocacy and education work with these agencies has been to identify steps that they can take to better serve the LGBT community. To accomplish this goal, the Foundation provides opportunities for Network members with particular kinds of expertise and backgrounds to meet with agency commissioners, directors, and program staff to educate, build relationships, and share information on the needs of the community. Extensive research is conducted by the Foundation in advance of these meetings on the mission and goals of the agencies, their budget, organizational and management structure, and previous efforts they have made to address the needs of LGBT individuals. Network participants meet beforehand with the Foundation to review the research, identify issues and the individuals responsible for addressing them, and to formulate the "ask" that the agency will be held accountable for delivering.

Steps that state agencies have taken in response to the collective efforts of the Foundation, Network and individual Network members include:

- The State Department of Health (DOH) issued an LGBT-inclusive Request for Proposals (RFP) in 1998 to distribute $1 million in grants under the Lesbian and Gay Health and Human Services Initiative. This was the first time that a New York State agency had identified LGBT people as an underserved population and established a mechanism to distribute government funds to address the community's needs. DOH issued a second RFP in 2002 to distribute $2.5 million in grants for LGBT health and human services.

- The State Office for the Aging (SOFA) included in its official planning document *Project 2015: The Future of Aging in New York State* a section devoted to the needs of LGBT senior citizens. This was the first time that any state agency had included LGBT people in an official long-range planning document.
- Following the lead of the Office of Alcoholism and Substance Abuse Services (OASAS), the Office for the Prevention of Domestic Violence (OPDV) developed a curriculum to train health and human service providers how to screen for domestic violence among LGBT clients and to understand this population's unique needs.
- By defining those of same-sexual orientation as an underserved population, the Division of Criminal Justice Services (DCJS) included LGBT victims of domestic violence in its implementation of the federal S.T.O.P. Violence Against Women Act.
- The State Education Department (SED) promulgated rules that required every public school district in the state to document and report acts of bias-related bullying, harassment, and intimidation, including anti-gay harassment.
- The Office of Children and Family Services (OCFS) expanded the number of Network organizations receiving grants for counseling, support and school violence prevention programs targeted to LGBT youth.

The Foundation and the Network are committed to the principle that affirming the sexuality and gender identity of LGBT individuals is a key to their mental health and well-being. To emphasize this in the area of mental health delivery for LGBT individuals with significant, chronic psychiatric disorders, the Foundation and Network advocate for the expansion and replication of unique public programs like the LGBT Affirmative Program for People with Major Mental Illness at the Heights Hill Mental Health Service of South Beach Psychiatric Center, operated by the State Office for Mental Health (OMH).

Legislative Advocacy

The Pride Agenda sponsors an annual Lobby Day during which members of the LGBT community from across the state come to Albany to advocate for the organization's legislative priorities, including the recently passed Sexual Orientation Non-Discrimination Act (SONDA), the Hate Crimes Act passed that passed in 2000, and the Dignity for All Students Act.

Recognizing the need to focus on a LGBT health and human services agenda, the Foundation began, in 1999, to organize separate meetings during

Lobby Day among the members of the Network and the chairs and staff of eight targeted New York State Assembly committees. These meetings were designed to provide an educational opportunity on the health and human service needs of the LGBT community, and to advocate for funding to support organizations that serve this community.

The Foundation selected those Assembly committees most closely related to the types of services that Network members were interested in providing to the community. They included: Aging; Alcohol and Drug Abuse; Children and Families; Codes, which has jurisdiction over hate crimes, domestic violence and sexual assault; Education; Health; Mental Health; and Social Services, which has jurisdiction over public assistance and homelessness.

Starting in 2001, the Network decided to establish a clear demarcation between lobbying on legislative issues and advocating for health and human services. It created a separate, stand-alone Advocacy Day for the Network. Similar to meetings scheduled on Lobby Day, Advocacy Day is held every year between the Governor's January submission of the Executive Budget to the State Assembly and Senate, and their deadline to pass a final budget by April 1st. During this critical time, Network members can urge legislators to include funding in the state budget for LGBT health and human services. Meetings have been expanded to include the legislative committees in the State Senate and the Ranking Minority members of committees in both houses of the State Legislature.

The planning for Advocacy Day requires a minimum of six months lead time to accomplish the following tasks: organizing a planning committee; agreeing on an agenda; choosing speakers and presentations; preparing a budget; identifying sources of financial support for Network travel, lodging, supplies and food; securing commitments from Network members to insure representation of the broadest range of issues, communities and geographic areas; preparing a training program designed to meet the needs of both experienced and first time advocates; selecting the legislative committees; scheduling appointments with the Assembly and Senate committee chairs, ranking Minority members and staff; preparing informational materials, such as fact sheets for the legislators, as well as voting records, meeting report and evaluation forms for the participants; matching participants with their preferred committee meetings; and designating meeting facilitators.

An important key to conducting effective legislative meetings is training participants in advance. A training curriculum was developed in 2002 that could be downloaded electronically, and used by individual Network members to train their staff, board and constituents. This curriculum is also used to conduct a half-day training in Albany on the day before Advocacy Day. It provides an explanation of the purpose of the Network and of Advocacy Day; the history of state funding of LGBT health and human services, the Governor's

Executive Budget, and the role of the State Legislature in passing the final state budget. It defines the role of constituents in advocating for their needs. It characterizes the targeted legislative committees and committee chairs, and the role of the group facilitator. It provides information on how to structure an effective meeting, and how to identify and train a group facilitator. Time is included for ample "role plays" of legislative meetings, developing a focus on the personal stories of individual participants, making the "ask," and getting a commitment from the legislator. An abbreviated version of the training is conducted on the morning of Advocacy Day for those individuals unable to participate in the prior day's training.

Following Advocacy Day, the Foundation coordinates its advocacy efforts with the Pride Agenda to support the funding requests made to the State Legislature. This involves asking Network members to send letters to their local Assembly Members and to the Assembly Speaker, scheduling in-district and face-to-face meetings with legislators, issuing e-mail alerts and sending a letter to the Assembly Speaker on behalf of the entire Network.

These advocacy efforts have had the following results:

1997

The governor and the state legislature included in the budget $1 million appropriated to DOH to fund community-based organizations across the state. These funds provided a range of non-HIV/AIDS specific services designed to promote wellness and access to health and human services for New York's lesbian and gay community. Late adoption of the budget and delay in issuing a Request for Proposals by DOH meant that none of the money for the initiative was spent at that time. Recognizing the importance of this funding, the state legislature passed a budget in 1998 which included an additional $1 million in funding plus a reappropriation of the unspent $1 million from state fiscal year 1997-1998. After directing DOH to issue the RFP, the Governor vetoed the entire $2 million. Letters and phone calls from lesbian, gay and straight New Yorkers, as well as legislators, led to the governor agreeing to make $1 million available in discretionary funding under the Lesbian and Gay Health and Human Services Initiative.

1998

Seventy-two organizations from all parts of the state submitted proposals for funding under the Lesbian and Gay Health and Human Services Initiative. In December, the Department of Health issued grants totaling $1 million to eleven groups across the state, 10 of which were members of the Network.

1999

Led by the Assembly Majority and the Assembly Speaker, the state legislature appropriated $2 million in the state fiscal year (SFY) 1999-2000 budget to DOH for programs designed to meet the non-HIV health and social service needs of LGBT populations. In February of 2000, $2 million in grants were issued to 27 groups (17 of which were Network members).

2000

Again led by the Assembly, the state legislature expanded funding by including $2.5 million in the SFY 2000-2001 budget for LGBT health and human services. In October of 2000, the Assembly Speaker announced that $2.5 million in grants would be issued to 39 groups (29 of which were Network members). Supported by the advocacy efforts of the Foundation and the Network, the Speaker committed to an additional $175,000 in state and federal monies to fund two additional Network members. Thus, over 40 community-based organizations, the majority of which were Network members, received grants that funded a variety of health and human service needs of LGBT New Yorkers, including youth, people of color, seniors and transgender individuals.

2001

LGBT community-based organizations received no new funding for health and human services in the SFY 2001-2002 budget because the state legislature passed a bare bones budget that excluded funding for non-profits. A supplemental budget passed by the state legislature several months later included a partial restoration of funding for non-profits across the state; however, LGBT provider organizations did not receive any grants out of that appropriation in 2001.

2002

The Assembly Speaker announced $1.5 million in grants to Network members out of the SFY 2001-2002 supplemental budget to partially restore what they had not received in the prior year. In January of 2002, the Governor fulfilled a promise he made in the fall of 2001 by including, for the first time in his Executive Budget, $2.5 million to fund Network organizations. In May of 2002, the state legislature passed the SFY 2002-2003 budget that included the Governor's $2.5 million in addition to $1.1 million appropriated by the Assembly Speaker. This funding, later increased by the Assembly Speaker to

$1.2 million, is the largest amount of funding that the Network has received to date in any single state budget.

CONCLUSION: WHAT NEXT?

The success of the Foundation's and Network's advocacy and education strategies can obscure the fact that, in contrast to the success of other culturally-based communities throughout New York State, the LGBT community is still in the early stages of developing, implementing and refining a coordinated and sophisticated strategy designed to insure that state government responds to its basic needs. The model of having social service providers articulate a need, but also flex political muscle, has reaped impressive results. However, the total amount of funding pales in comparison to the health and human service needs of the LGBT community.

The report on Lesbian, Gay, Bisexual and Transgender Health: Finding and Concerns issued by the Gay and Lesbian Medical Association and the Columbia University Joseph L. Mailman School of Public Health in 2000 noted that "In mental health care, stigma, lack of cultural sensitivity, and unconscious and conscious reluctance to address sexuality may all hamper effectiveness of care." This assessment is also true of the care of LGBT people struggling with alcohol and substance abuse, domestic violence, poor health, harassment in school, and homelessness, as well as those seniors living in nursing homes.

To address these needs, the next phase of the Foundation's and Network's advocacy and education efforts in partnership with the Pride Agenda will focus not only on expanding funding in the state budget, but also on making sure that state agencies: (a) assume diversity in sexual orientation and provide staff training on sexuality, including sexual orientation and gender identity, and integrate this training with ongoing multi-cultural training efforts; and (b) target agency services to LGBT individuals and institutionalize LGBT issues and concerns throughout the entire agency and provider agencies.

NOTES

1. The Sexual Orientation Non-Discrimination Act (SONDA) that bans discrimination on the basis of sexual orientation in housing, employment, public accommodations, education and credit was passed by the State Legislature and signed into law by Governor Pataki on December 17, 2002 effective January 16, 2003.

2. Terminology used in this article reflects the evolution of community identity from primarily lesbian and gay to a more inclusive lesbian, gay, bisexual and transgender (LGBT).

3. Request for Proposals issued March 20, 1998 by the New York State Department of Health.

4. State of the State Report 1999; Lesbian and Gay New Yorkers and Their Families.

5. State of the State Report 2000; Building Community Assets: Lesbian, Gay, Transgender and Bisexual New Yorkers and Their Families.

6. State of the State Report 2001; New York State and the Lesbian, Gay, Bisexual and Transgendered Community: Profiles of a Partnership.

REFERENCES

Empire State Pride Agenda Foundation, State of the State Report 1999; *Lesbian and Gay New Yorkers and Their Families.*

Empire State Pride Agenda Foundation, State of the State Report 2000; *Building Community Assets: Lesbian, Gay, Transgender and Bisexual New Yorkers and Their Families.*

Empire State Pride Agenda Foundation, State of the State Report 2001; *New York State and the Lesbian, Gay, Bisexual and Transgendered Community: Profiles of a Partnership.*

New York State Department of Health, Request for Proposals, March 20, 1998.

APPENDIX

Members of the New York State Lesbian, Gay, Bisexual and Transgender
Health and Human Services Network

African Ancestral Lesbians United for Societal Change
c/o The Center
1 Little West 12th Street
New York, NY 10014
212-620-7310
www.aalusc.org
Committed to the spiritual, cultural, educational, economic and social empowerment of African ancestral lesbians and women of color living in New York
City. Provides educational tools, resources and referrals, workshops and discussions, and social and cultural events.

Asian Women Healing Ourselves
34-10 75th Street, #6K
Jackson Heights, NY 11372
A coalition of Asian and Pacific Islander women dedicated to addressing the
health concerns of Asian and Pacific Islander lesbians and bisexual women in
the New York City area.

Audre Lorde Project
85 South Oxford Street
Brooklyn, NY 11217
718-596-0342
www.alp.org
A community organizing center for lesbian, gay, bisexual, two-spirit and
transgender people of color communities. Through mobilization, education
and capacity building, ALP works for community wellness and progressive
social/economic justice by and for people of African/Black/Caribbean, Arab,
Asian and Pacific Islander, Latino/a and Native/Indigenous descent.

Aya Institute
c/o Audre Lorde Project
85 South Oxford Street
Brooklyn, NY 11217
A group of people of African descent in New York City dedicated to education
and spiritual and mental health.

Bronx Lesbian & Gay Health Resource Consortium
940 Garrison Avenue
Bronx, NY 10474
718-842-9831
blghrc@aol.com
Provides a database and directory of health care and social service providers
who are informed of and sensitive to the LGBT community in the Bronx.

Callen-Lorde Community Health Center
356 West 18th Street
New York, NY 10011
212-271-7200
www.callen-lorde.org
A full-service, state-licensed health center geared primarily to the LGBT community, including those living with HIV. Services include comprehensive primary and specialty medical care, mental health care and health education. All
services provided regardless of ability to pay.

Capital District Gay and Lesbian Community Council
P.O. Box 131
Albany, NY 12201
518-462-6138
cdglcc@aol.com
www.cdglcc.org
Serves the Capital District's gay, lesbian, bisexual and transgender community. The Council seeks to promote understanding and acceptance of the
LGBT community and to provide important programs and services to the community.

Center for Crime Victim and Sexual Assault Services of Tompkins County
(CVSA)
408 West State Street
Ithaca, NY 14850
607-273-5589
www.cvsa-tc.org
Works to reduce incidences of sexual assault, abuse and harassment in
Tompkins County through educational programming and advocacy. Provides
crisis response and counseling services for rape and sexual assault survivors
and their families and friends.

Center Lane/Westchester Jewish Community Services
845 North Broadway, Suite 2
White Plains, NY 10603
914-948-1042
centerlane@hotmail.com
Located in Westchester County, Center Lane offers a drop-in center, discussion groups, social activities, a peer leadership program and individual and family counseling for LGBT youth. Its services are utilized by adolescents from Westchester, Putnam, Rockland and the Bronx.

Colombian Lesbian and Gay Association (COLEGA)
35-15 Leverich Street, Suite 607
Jackson Heights, NY 11372
(718) 670-7399
colega_ny@yahoo.com
www.colegalgbt.org
Advocates for the health, visibility, voice and strength of all immigrant LGBT Colombians. COLEGA has linkages with LGBT advocacy organizations in Colombia, South America.

Community Awareness Network for a Drug-Free Life and Environment (CANDLE)
120 North Main Street, Suite 301
New City, NY 10956-5188
845-634-6677
http: //209.68.1.37/web/candle/
Works to prevent the abuse of alcohol and other drugs by Rockland County youth through programs that build resiliency, educate about health and sexuality issues and help youth cope with stress due to peer, school or family problems.

Gay & Lesbian Switchboard of Long Island
34 West Main Street
Bay Shore, NY 11706
631-665-3700
www.glsbli.com
Serves as a source of information, referral and peer counseling for residents of Long Island by telephone weeknights 7-10 p.m.

Gay & Lesbian Youth Services of Western New York
190 Franklin Street
Buffalo, NY 14202
716-855-0221
www.glyswny.com

Provides programming for youth ages 14-21 from Niagara and Erie counties. They provide a safe and positive environment for lesbian, gay, bisexual, transgender and questioning (LGBTQ) youth to learn more about themselves through peer interaction and educational experiences. The organization creates opportunities for emotional growth and community awareness.

Gay Alliance of the Genesee Valley
179 Atlantic Avenue
Rochester, NY 14607
585-244-8640
info@gayalliance.org
www.gayalliance.org
The only LGBT agency in Monroe County and the outlying area, GAGV serves approximately 15,000 people a year through its support groups, recreational programming, information and referral hotline, publications and sensitivity outreach trainings.

Gay and Lesbian Coalition of Western New York
206 S. Elmwood Avenue
Buffalo, NY 14201
716-847-0315
Works to make Western New York a safe, healthy and enriched place for LGBT people to live, work and establish their families. Identifies community needs, strengthens communication and educates the public about the value that LGBT people add to society.

Gay, Lesbian and Straight Education Network (GLSEN)
121 West 27th Street, Suite 804
New York, NY 10001
212-727-0135
glsen@glsen.org
www.glsen.org
An organization of teachers, parents, students and concerned citizens working together to end anti-gay bias in schools. GLSEN has over 85 grassroots chapters across the country, including five in New York (Albany, Hudson Valley, Long Island, New York City and Rochester).

Gay Men of African Descent (GMAD)
103 East 125th Street, Suite 503
New York, NY 10035
212-828-1697
gmad@aol.com
www.gmad.org

Works to empower gay men of African descent through education, social support, political advocacy and health and wellness promotion. Programs include HIV prevention through street and community outreach, discussion and support groups, a drop-in center and capacity-building assistance services.

Gay Men's Health Crisis
119 West 24th Street
New York, NY 10011
212-367-1000
www.gmhc.org
Founded by volunteers in 1981, GMHC is the oldest and largest not-for-profit AIDS organization in the United States, offering hands-on support services, education and advocacy.
Greater Utica Lambda Fellowship (GULF)
P.O. Box 122
Utica, NY 13503
Encompassing the counties of Oneida, Herkimer and Madison, GULF provides outreach and support to gay and lesbian people in a safe and supportive environment.

Griot Circle
30 Third Avenue
Brooklyn, NY 11217
718-246-2775
An intergenerational and culturally diverse Brooklyn-based organization providing social services and support programs for older lesbian, gay, bisexual, transgender and two-spirit people of color.

Heights-Hill Mental Health Service
South Beach Psychiatric Center
LesBiGay & Transgender Affirmative Program
25 Flatbush Avenue, 3rd Floor
Brooklyn, NY 11217
718-875-1420
Located in downtown Brooklyn, the LGBT Affirmative Program provides sensitive, professional services for LGBT individuals with major mental illness.

Hetrick Martin Institute
2 Astor Place
New York, NY 10003
212-674-2400
www.hmi.org

HMI creates a safe and supportive environment for lesbian, gay, bisexual, transgender and questioning youth between the ages of 12 and 21 and their families. Through a comprehensive package of direct services and referrals, HMI seeks to foster healthy youth development. It serves thousands of LGBT youth and their families each month from all five boroughs of New York City and the surrounding metropolitan area.

In Our Own Voices
33 Central Avenue
Albany, NY 12202
518-432-4188
A collaborative effort of four community-based organizations, IOOV's mission is to promote and ensure the physical, mental, spiritual, political, social, cultural and economic health and survival of LGBT people of color communities in the Capital District.

Institute for Human Identity
160 West 24th Street
New York, NY 10011
212-243-2830
www.altrue.net/site/therapycenter
Provides professional counseling and psychotherapy services to the LGBT community in an affirmative environment. Trains mental health professionals and offers public forums on how best to address the psychological needs of the LGBT community.

Lambda Treatment and Recovery Program
87-08 Justice Avenue, Suite 1-G
Elmhurst, NY 11373
718-476-8480
Part of the Human Service Centers, a state-licensed facility with over 20 years of experience in the field of addictions and mental health. Professionals specialize in LGBT-sensitive crisis intervention, substance abuse, addictions, relapse prevention and behavioral health management.

Lavender Lamps
740 Riverside Drive, Apt. 1K
New York, NY 10031
A New York City-based organization for LGBT nurses, offering support, discussion groups and a newsletter.

Lesbian and Gay Family Building Project/Ferre Institute
124 Front Street
Binghamton, NY 13905
607-724-4308
LesGayFamBldg@aol.com
www.ferre.org
Provides family building information to members of the lesbian and gay community in upstate New York, including information on adoptions, donor insemination, surrogacy and foster care.

Long Island Gay and Lesbian Youth (LIGALY)
34 Park Avenue
Bay Shore, NY 11706
631-665-2300
www.ligaly.com
LIGALY provides counseling services, a drop-in center, support groups and social and recreational activities for lesbian and gay youth and their families in Nassau and Suffolk counties.

Mano a Mano
c/o Latino Commission on AIDS
24 West 25th Street, 9th Floor
New York, NY 10010-2704
212-584-9311
mano_mano_ny@hotmail.com
A network of New York City-based Latino LGBT organizations and activists that advocates for health and social services issues affecting New York's Latino LGBT community, disseminates information on activities and services available to this community, and offers technical support and assistance to emerging Latino LGBT organizations.

Men of Color Health Awareness
25 Franklin Street, Suite 1060
Rochester, NY 14604
585-420-1400
Provides services to men of color who have sex with men. The services include, but are not limited to: HIV/AIDS education, prevention, outreach, case management, support groups and community building activities.

Metropolitan Community Church of NY
446 West 36th Street
New York, NY 10018
212-629-7440
www.mccny.org

Provides worship services, pastoral care, an HIV/AIDS nutrition program, emergency food programs, support groups and other services. Seeks to minister to the spiritual and physical needs of the LGBT community. A member of the Universal Fellowship of Metropolitan Community Churches.

New Neutral Zone
12 East 33rd Street, 10th Floor
New York, NY 10016
646-935-1943
A drop-in center for LGBT youth and their straight allies ages 15-22. Offers counseling, recreation, peer outreach and leadership, and arts programming in a youth-directed space.

New York City Gay and Lesbian Anti-Violence Project
240 West 35th Street, Suite 200
New York, NY 10001
212-714-1184
webmaster@avp.org
www.avp.org
Assists LGBT and HIV-affected survivors of hate-motivated violence, domestic violence, sexual assault and police misconduct by providing therapeutic counseling, advocacy within the criminal justice system and victim support agencies, information for self-help and referrals to practicing professionals.

People of Color in Crisis
468 Bergen Street
Brooklyn, NY 11217
718-230-0770
poccgen@pocc.org
Health and mental health services, including education, discussion, outreach and support, for the African-American and Caribbean LGBT communities.

Planned Parenthood of Niagara County
752 Portage Road
Niagara Falls, NY 14301
716-205-0704
Provides high quality, confidential reproductive and complementary health care services, educational programs promoting safe and responsible sexual attitudes and behavior, and advocacy for public policies reflecting these services.

Pride Community Center of Central New York
P.O. Box 6608
Syracuse, NY 13217
315-476-8006
pridesyrny@aol.com
www.cnypride.org
An all-volunteer organization offering a variety of programs for LGBT people in Central New York.

Pride for Youth: Long Island Crisis Center
2050 Bellmore Avenue
Bellmore, NY 11710
516-679-9000
www.licrisiscenter.org/pride.html
Provides an array of health and wellness services for LGBT youth in Nassau and Suffolk counties, including crisis counseling, support groups and recreational activities.

Pride Senior Network
132 West 22nd Street, 4th Floor
New York, NY 10011
212-675-1941
psn@pridesenior.org
www.pridesenior.org
Through advocacy, education and communication, encourages and promotes services that foster the health, well-being and quality of life for the aging LGBT population. Publishes an aging issues newspaper and service provider directory.

Queens Rainbow Community Center
P.O. Box 580445
Flushing, NY 11358
718-457-2928
Disseminates information about LGBT communities to foster knowledge and understanding. Educates the public, creates/supports activities commemorating important LGBT historical events and creates/supports social service programs that improve the health and wellness of LGBT people, their families and friends.

Queens Pride House
67-03 Woodside Avenue
Woodside, NY 11377
718-429-5309
queenspridehouse.tripod.com

Provides a safe, nurturing space for the Queens LGBT community, including an expansive library of publications and videos. Services include community building, education both inside and outside the community and increasing political awareness.

Rainbow Access Initiative
200 Henry Johnson Boulevard
Albany, NY 12210
518-471-9080
rainbowaccess.org
Addresses the educational needs of medical and social service professionals regarding the health and human service issues of the LGBT community by training non-LGBT health and human service professionals and empowering LGBT health care consumers.

SAGE Queens
74-09 37th Avenue, Room 409
Jackson Heights, NY 11372
718-533-6469
Provides recreation, socialization, education, organizing and referrals for LGBT senior citizens in Queens.

SAGE/Upstate
P.O. Box 6271
Syracuse, NY 13217
315-446-1319
Provides recreational, social and educational programming for aging LGBT people in Onandaga and contiguous counties.

Seamen's Society for Children and Families
Supportive Services Clinic
25 Hyatt Street
Staten Island, NY 10301-2321
718-447-7740
http: //community.silive.com/cc/rootsandwings
Mental health clinic administered by the Seamen's Society that provides free mental health services to the LGBT community.

Senior Action in a Gay Environment (SAGE)
305 Seventh Avenue, 16th Floor
New York, NY 10001
212-741-2247
sageusa@aol.com

A social service and advocacy agency for older members of the LGBT community. Provides over 300 opportunities for socialization each month and an extensive program of education and community outreach. Located in New York City, with affiliates throughout the country.

Shades of Lavender
c/o Brooklyn AIDS Task Force
502 Bergen Street
Brooklyn, NY 11217
718-622-2910
A multicultural space in Brooklyn created by and for the lesbian and bisexual women's community. Provides ongoing discussion and self-help groups, workshops, activities and information and referrals for youth and adults.

The LGBT Community Center
208 West 13th Street
New York, NY 10011
212-620-7310
webmaster@gaycenter.org
www.gaycenter.org
Serving New York City's LGBT community since 1983. More than 5,000 people each week access the Center's mental health, family, substance abuse, HIV/AIDS-related, educational, cultural, advocacy and recreational services.

The LOFT
180 East Post Road, Lower Level
White Plains, NY 10601
914-948-2932
www.loftgaycenter.org
Serves over 3,000 LGBT people each month in the lower Hudson Valley. Offers support groups, a newsletter, a telephone helpline, and social, educational and recreational programming.

Unity Fellowship Church
230 Classon Avenue
Brooklyn, NY 11205
718-636-5646
http://members.aol.com/ufcnyc/
Located in Brooklyn, Unity provides education and support services for LGBT people ages 18 to 25 and their families.

Women-Oriented Women
1005 Brayton Park Place
Utica, NY 13502
315-735-9704
www.borg.com/~berta/
A Utica-based lesbian organization, holding monthly social meetings and recreational activities.

A Program for Lesbian, Gay, Bisexual, and Transgender Individuals with Major Mental Illness

Ronald E. Hellman, MD
Eileen Klein, PhD

SUMMARY. This paper reports on The LGBT Affirmative Program of South Beach Psychiatric Center, a public sector mental health program in New York State for lesbian, gay, bisexual, and transgender (LGBT) individuals with major mental illness. The program began in 1996 and has provided services to over 200 individuals as of June, 2004. Systemic and cultural factors influencing program development are described. Evolution of the program components are summarized. A survey sampling psychiatric patients/clients who attended the program in May, 2000 demonstrated a high level of satisfaction with the services offered. The program is viewed as an important resource to the clinic and the community. *[Article copies available for a fee from The Haworth Document Delivery Service: 1-800-HAWORTH. E-mail address: <docdelivery@haworthpress. com> Website: <http://www.HaworthPress.com> © 2004 by The Haworth Press, Inc. All rights reserved.]*

Ronald E. Hellman is Program Director for the Affirmative Program, South Beach Psychiatric Center, 25 Flatbush Avenue, 3rd Floor, Brooklyn, NY 11217 (E-mail: SBOPREH@gw.omh.state.ny.us).

Eileen Klein is Chief of Services at the Heights Hill Mental Health Service, South Beach Psychiatric Center.

The authors wish to thank Christian Huygens, PhD, for assistance organizing the consumer survey, Jean Okie, PhD, and Lori Gralnick, CSW, for comments on the manuscript, and Maya Iwata for her assistance regarding the Rainbow Heights Club.

[Haworth co-indexing entry note]: "A Program for Lesbian, Gay, Bisexual, and Transgender Individuals with Major Mental Illness." Hellman, Ronald E., and Eileeen Klein. Co-published simultaneously in *Journal of Gay & Lesbian Psychotherapy* (The Haworth Medical Press, an imprint of The Haworth Press, Inc.) Vol. 8, No. 3/4, 2004, pp. 67-82; and: *Handbook of LGBT Issues in Community Mental Health* (ed: Ronald E. Hellman, and Jack Drescher) The Haworth Medical Press, an imprint of The Haworth Press, Inc., 2004, pp. 67-82. Single or multiple copies of this article are available for a fee from The Haworth Document Delivery Service [1-800-HAWORTH, 9:00 a.m. - 5:00 p.m. (EST). E-mail address: docdelivery@haworthpress.com].

Digital Object Identifer: 10.1300/J236v08n03_05

KEYWORDS. Bisexual, cultural diversity, gay, homosexuality, lesbian, mental illness, mental health services, psychiatric disorder, public psychiatry, sexual minorities, transgender

INTRODUCTION

While there is now a considerable body of literature on the psychological concerns of sexual minority individuals (Cabaj and Stein, 1996), little has been written about culturally relevant mental health services for those of variant sexual and gender orientations with major psychiatric disorders (McCarn, 1999). This paper describes the evolution of a culturally focused program for lesbian, gay, bisexual, and transgender (LGBT) individuals with severe and disabling forms of psychiatric disorder who receive treatment in a mainstream, public mental health center.

The LGBT Affirmative Program of South Beach Psychiatric Center (SBPC) began in February, 1996 with the goal of providing culturally relevant services to sexual minority individuals with severe and persistent psychiatric disorders. The provision of effective psychiatric services to culturally diverse populations is an area of significant contemporary concern in the mental health field. The National Mental Health Association and the Joint Commission on Accreditation of Healthcare Organizations have identified the provision of culturally competent mental health treatment as essential to delivering relevant services that are clinically effective and cost effective (Graham, 1998).

The development of these services can be a challenging task. Culturally focused service provision must include an awareness by mental health professionals of clients' unique psycho-social and treatment needs that derive from their cultural background, as well as the interpersonal dynamics related to the cultural group identifications and customs that operate between the recipients of mental health services and those responsible for their care. Clinicians and administrators must then translate this knowledge into meaningful policies and interventions at all levels of service delivery (Aponte, Rivers and Wohl, 1995).

HISTORICAL BACKGROUND

In a state midway between reason and madness, those afflicted were in constant danger of becoming insane and thus required the protection of the asylum.

(Ronald Bayer, 1981, p.19)

The psychiatric categorization of homosexuality for more than a century resulted in its inclusion, along with psychotic, affective, anxiety, and other disorders, within the domain of mental illnesses. Major mental illness typically refers to more severe and disabling forms of psychiatric disorder, lasting for many years, often associated with psychiatric hospitalizations and significant functional disability (Soreff, 1996). By this definition, few would have classified homosexuality as a major mental illness. Nevertheless, in a 19th century view, as Bayer notes above, some were convinced otherwise.

A prevailing belief among some psychiatric authorities was that homosexuality (and major psychiatric disorders) occurred in very troubled heterosexual persons (Lewes, 1988). Clinical objectives in that era included investigation of the etiology of these disorders so that appropriate treatments could be developed in order to bring about a sound, heterosexual life.

Such views were initially challenged from outside the field of psychiatry (Bayer, 1981). Kinsey (1948, 1953), Ford and Beach (1951), and Hooker (1957) demonstrated that homosexuality was not rare, marginal, or pathological. They, and others, revealed how methodological problems resulted in false generalizations about homosexuality, by recognizing that studies were generalizing from small numbers of clinical and prison samples. Pathologizing views were inevitably confronted by psychiatrists, as clinicians like Szasz (1974) and Marmor (1965) demonstrated how diverse identities and behaviors could be confused with diagnoses, and how cultural values could influence psychiatric classification.

Concurrently, a new cultural subgroup was emerging in the social arena. The Stonewall riots of June, 1969 marked the transition of an underground homosexual subculture to a new, openly gay minority. The former, steeped in secrecy in response to being pathologized, stigmatized, and criminalized, now candidly struggled to overcome oppressive attitudes, biases, and stereotypes. As acceptance grew, this counter-cultural group eventually took its place within the larger, sanctioned multi-cultural milieu.

These changes demanded a shift in clinical focus. In the 1970s, multi-disciplinary challenges to the illness model of homosexuality resulted in the emergence of affirmative constructs of gay/lesbian mental health. These stood in contrast to the change-oriented therapies that had preceded them which devalued non-heterosexual desire. Efforts to help sexual minority individuals cope with disparaging social attitudes, and find affiliations within an affirming community, replaced interventions to eliminate homosexuality.

Affirmative treatment approaches first developed in so-called alternative treatment centers rooted in philosophies and organizational structures that challenged the heterosexual orthodoxy of mainstream agencies (Gonsiorek, 1982). Grass-roots treatment centers, however, lacked the experience and infrastructure to manage patients suffering from serious and persistent mental illness. Sexual minority individuals with major psychiatric disorders had little choice but to remain in mainstream settings.

Thus, gay people with major mental illness continued to find themselves in a cultural limbo. Gay pride could not overcome the stigma of mental illness. Those with major psychiatric disorders continued to experience a lack of acceptance from within the gay community, while finding limited tolerance from the psychiatric community because of their sexual orientation.

THE CONTEMPORARY CHALLENGE

Mainstream psychiatric settings have not routinely provided for the sociocultural needs of those with a homosexual or cross-gender identity. In more recent years, as perspective on cultural issues in psychiatry has grown, the cultural relevance of existing public sector mental health programs has come into question regarding LGBT populations. A 1998 survey of 100 NYC funded mental health agencies found, for example, that 93% did not have any specific LGBT services (Lesbian, Gay, Bisexual, Transgender Mental Hygiene Issues Committee, 1998).

One reason for the lack of culturally relevant services may be that the majority of patients seen in mainstream clinical settings are not gay/transgender, so that assessing the particular circumstances and needs of LGBT individuals tends not to be as routine, nor is there a high demand for such services. Societal recognition of LGBT individuals as members of a legitimate subculture is barely decades old, and the incorporation of culturally relevant programming for sexual minorities is only beginning to find its place in the mainstream mental health setting.

Another reason may have to do with the influence of the established psychiatric subculture in the mental health setting. Public institutions providing mental health services are historically rooted in approaches that did not address the person with chronic psychiatric disability from a cultural perspective. Culturally affirmative programming, therefore, requires reconstruction of existing programming, and this has been slow to develop. Lingering professional ambivalence, cultural estrangement of the mainstream from this minority group, and generic factors, such as resistance to organizational change, may all contribute to the current widespread deficit.

A CULTURAL EDUCATION

In 1995, the Heights Hill Mental Health Service of South Beach Psychiatric Center in New York began to look more closely at its own cultural vantage as a public, mainstream mental health institution. Treatment experience with those from diverse backgrounds, including sexual minority individuals, confirmed that most clinicians, patients, and ancillary staff in this setting were heterosexual. Talks with known LGBT clients established that they tended to perceive the community mental health center (CMHC) as a "heterosexual" institution. LGBT clients tended to feel less safe, were less open, expected less of a focus on LGBT issues, and were more subject to heterosexism, homophobia, and transphobia (Hellman, 1996).

It was acknowledged that viewing LGBT clients as potential members of a cultural minority group within the clinic had been significantly overlooked. What emerged was an understanding that LGBT clients adapt to the CMHC setting, but typically do not identify with it as an LGBT cultural resource. There was virtually no opportunity for sexual minority group cohesion to occur in the mental health service, and this seemed true, in general, for public sector treatment facilities.

It followed that when the mainstream, public sector clinic does not recognize itself as a "heterosexual" cultural institution, or superficially defines itself as an "integrated" setting, it tends not to facilitate development of a context or service provision that can nurture sexual minority cultural identity. Sexual minority individuals with chronic psychiatric problems are left to adapt to a heterosexual environment regardless of their level of cultural sexual identity. This may foster limited personal development and lessen the patient/client's ability to be authentic within the psychiatric subculture. The cultural context of sexual identity is important in its own right, but for those with major mental illness, the possibility that a shared cultural sexual identity, fostered and integrated within the mental health setting, could provide a salubrious counterbalance to long entrenched psychiatric identities and roles was more reason to initiate a program.

Further discussion suggested that the dominant cultural group in the clinic, as defined by heterosexual identity, was not aware that LGBT patients participated in relation to it. The groups coexisted within the CMHC, but the LGBT proto-community had no "space" of its own. There were no LGBT activities, no LGBT signifiers, no LGBT groups and, therefore, no opportunity for LGBT people with mental disabilities to nurture a cultural identity as members of a sexual minority community within the mental health service environment. Nor were there opportunities for the dominant client group to process issues related to their sexual minority peers. While differing values, concerns, and conflicts between those of dissimilar sexual identities were sometimes articulated and addressed in the generic mental health setting, many opportunities for the cultural growth of sexual identity were lost.

THE LGBT PSYCHIATRIC CLIENT

LGBT individuals often arrive in the mainstream psychiatric setting either involuntarily, or because the services they need do not exist in the LGBT community, or because they have limited financial choices. The LGBT patient often has problems obtaining financial resources since their ability to work is compromised both by functional disability, and the stigma of psychiatric disability and sexual minority status. This dual stigma often prevents members of this group from availing themselves of employment opportunities, and complicates obtaining entitlements, such as Medicaid, which could pay for needed mental health services in clinics that require a fee-for-service. The LGBT client may be treated differently in social service agencies, as well, and may need additional staff support to apply for benefits for which they are eligible, such as supervised or subsidized housing. Something they have in common with others having major psychiatric disorders, is that they tend to be high utilizers of a multitude of mental health and social services and have difficulty fitting into the community. Their mental illness can disenfranchise them from their own cultural community, since few in the LGBT community have experienced serious psychiatric symptoms and disabilities. Nor have most members of the LGBT community experienced the world of inpatient units, day programs, residential placements, unemployment, and dependency on caregivers.

Sexual minority patients with psychiatric disabilities may have serious difficulty finding people with whom they can identify. They may be reluctant to reach out, and when they do, they tend to find limited support and scarce resources in the LGBT community. Their families also have difficulty finding relevant psychiatric services as they contend with both the psychiatric illness and sexual minority status of the family member.

THE PROGRAM AT SOUTH BEACH PSYCHIATRIC CENTER

The LGBT Affirmative Program is based at the Heights Hill Mental Health Service, one of seven outpatient clinics of SBPC, located in downtown Brooklyn, New York. SBPC is a CMHC governed and funded by the New York State Office of Mental Health (OMH). It serves a low-income, Medicaid eligible, urban, ethnically mixed population of various educational levels. As of June 2004, over 200 individuals have participated in the Program as one component of their broader psychiatric treatment. To the best of the authors' knowledge, prior to the establishment of this service, there were no other existing services in the New York metropolitan area for low-income, Medicaid/Medicare-eligible LGBT individuals with major mental illness.

The concept for the program took shape in response to SBPC's growing emphasis on the provision of culturally competent mental health services. This transpired as the mandate to recognize and address this fundamental domain matured. The National Mental Health Association, for example, now identifies culturally competent mental health treatment services as a "prerequisite for ethical and accurate assessment" (National Mental Health Association, 1999).

The administration and staff of the Heights Hill Mental Health Outpatient service met in 1995 to identify gaps in multi-cultural services. It was noted that there were specific programs directed at meeting the needs of Latinos, African-American and women patients, but a lack of services to the mentally ill LGBT client. A plan was outlined to develop relevant services within the context of SBPC's mainstream focus and within the Center's guidelines.

A heterogeneous group of interested staff formed a study group. The group's mission was to evaluate and clarify LGBT service needs and establish new program components within the fiscal limitations of a public health organization. Financial considerations initially prohibited the hiring of new staff for the proposed program. Space limitations, and restrictions in program support and supplies also lead to modest but workable solutions.

Most of the services provided by SBPC are catchment-area based, but because of the unique nature of this program, and the lower prevalence of this subgroup, it was decided to expand the geographical region served to include the entire NYC metropolitan area. It was agreed that heterosexual status would not preclude staff participation, but clinicians had to be reasonably knowledgeable and comfortable with the cross-cultural considerations, and willing to expand their horizons. Program ideas had to be presented to South Beach Psychiatric Center's central administration for approval before any plans could be implemented. In addition, any program ideas would have to be carried out within the guidelines of the NYS OMH.

With these considerations in mind, the study group formulated a program proposal that was presented to the Heights Hill clinical staff for feedback. Staff expressed concerns about why a new program was needed, why sexual orientation and gender variation should be considered cultural issues, why such a program should be given priority in a climate of downsizing and managed care, and how this would effect other culturally focused programs currently functioning at Heights Hill. These concerns were addressed with the staff before the proposal was presented to the SBPC administration for approval. Once authorization was received, the study group was dissolved and a steering committee formed to oversee the program.

Some early issues addressed by this committee included administration and staff conflict between their role as mental health "experts" and their level of comfort providing a new culturally focused service for which they might feel uninformed, inexperienced, and unaccustomed (Leigh, 1998); differing levels of interest for the new program; how to work with existing staff trained in traditional settings; disclosure of sexual identity to LGBT patients by staff; and concerns about the level of acceptance of non-LGBT staff by LGBT clients.

Self-disclosure, for example, at both patient activities and LGBT network meetings was an issue for staff. A heterosexual staff member presumed that others thought she was gay as a result of her involvement in the program. She was able to explore her thoughts and feelings about this in the committee meetings, and then developed an approach to disclosure that could enhance clients' and colleagues' perceptions of what it means to characterize others in terms of sexual identity, while discerning attributes that would be most essential or helpful to them in clinical work and program objectives.

Compliance and effective treatment rests on the ability to maintain oneself in a safe treatment community setting. There was an awareness that homophobic remarks were tolerated, for example, in the day program, inpatient units, and various residential settings. How likely was it that LGBT patients would continue to attend, find satisfaction with the treatment provided, and sustain a commitment to the necessary long-term treatments needed for effectively alleviating symptoms in such an environment (Graham, 1998)? Efforts would have to focus on incorporating attitudes and skills that were much more sensitive to this reality. It was also clear that the development of cultural competency in clinical work with this unique and heterogeneous group of mental health clients would be an ongoing process. The new program began with the understanding that expertise would increase with time and experience.

An openly gay staff member offered to serve as a consultant. A social work intern revealed she was a lesbian woman and, with a non-gay male therapist, volunteered to co-lead an LGBT support group. Staff were encouraged to "learn and do" together with input from LGBT patients directly, and through an ad hoc consumer advisory panel. A parallel process developed for patients and staff for self-disclosure and openness about their sexuality as a result of the new cross-cultural dialogue.

Staff interest in a training program led to the development of a speaker series to further develop clinical skills, awareness, and insight. Over time, more staff participated in this on-going in-service educational program as interest increased. During LGBT Pride Week in June each year, an LGBT film and discussion was presented in the Day Hospital for non-LGBT identified clients.

LGBT program materials were displayed in an effort to provide a safe, open milieu in which this minority could more comfortably begin to integrate its own culture into the mental health treatment setting. Affirmative posters and brochures describing the program were placed in the waiting room and day treatment community room to help overcome issues of taboo and secrecy, provide information, and create a more culturally friendly environment. Announcements of groups and activities were posted in the clinic and elevators, and reading materials were placed in the waiting room.

As a public agency, the Heights Hill Mental Health Service cannot receive private funding contributions. The service has an active Community Advisory Board that functions as a liaison between the Service and the community. The Board is a non-profit corporation made up of community members. The Board meets to discuss and inform the center of emerging community issues and explores cooperative ways to address these issues. In response to efforts by the Steering Committee, Heights Hill has been able to obtain corporate donations and grant funding through the Board.

A wide range of client needs were encountered as the program developed. Client interest resulted in the development of a cultural awareness group that focused on historical and cultural issues of relevance to the LGBT community, a reading room to help patients stay connected with outside issues, a monthly coffee klatch to enhance socialization, a newsletter, and a yearly LGBT Pride Party. The LGBT consumer advisory group decided to rename the program "Rainbow Heights" to further establish its own identity.

Affiliations were formed with other LGBT clinical agencies and adjunctive support facilities, and a staff member served as a liaison to the Empire State Pride Agenda, an advocacy and educational organization that backs funding initiatives on the state level. Interested psychology and social work students enabled the program to expand to include a transgender support group and additional social events such as a monthly LGBT movie night.

In September, 2002, the Rainbow Heights Club opened as a component of the Rainbow Heights program. This is an advocacy and empowerment based psychosocial program for LGBT adults with serious and persistent mental illness. Club members participate in social and vocational activities that include learning to prepare and provide meals for the club, computer training, digital photography and video, a newsletter, career and relationship groups, as well as a men's, women's, and transgender group.

The inherent complexity of cases required special attention. A homogenous "sexual minority" would soon be seen for its diversity, and sometimes clashing subgroups. Conflict would arise between those who were gender atypical, such as transgender clients, and those of conventional gender identity, those of different racial and ethnic backgrounds, lesbian women and gay men with culturally polarized gender dissimilarities, and those with different religious attitudes and levels of family support. All would interact with varied degrees of psychiatric symptoms, disability, levels of personality development, and psychological residue from disorders that could recur or remit at any time. Occasionally, a member of the support group would have to be excluded when these factors threatened the integrity of the group.

The LGBT support group demonstrated its fluency in the language of psychiatric experience to good therapeutic effect. Some members, for example, had a remarkable intuition for the line between healthy suspicion in the face of homophobia, and paranoia stemming from internal psychotic processes. As peers, they had more personal leverage with each other, and could confront, discuss, and clarify differences and concerns, often with a positive therapeutic outcome. Evolving subgroups kindled a process of exploration of internalized stereotypes and biases both within these sub-clusters, and in relation to the prevailing institutional subculture.

As the program became established, some of the more guarded, and demoralized patients appeared to become more comfortable and emotionally communicative. In some cases, it was apparent that their initial presentation, easily confused with the consequences of mental illness, had been significantly influenced by histories of adverse and limiting cross-cultural experiences that were exacerbated by an institutional transference. The new program framework, the relationship with a clinician affiliated with the program, and the new support of peers, all appeared to facilitate the ability to work through underlying defenses that had been necessary in the traditional setting.

For example, the staff's clinical impression of a patient with severe schizophrenia, due to a chronically blunted affect, was modified when this client became more related and expressive with treatment in the program. Although some residual blunting, characteristic of schizophrenia, remained, it became clear that emotional distancing and distrust secondary to alienation from the heterosexual mainstream and the larger gay community, had also played a significant role in this person's ability to relate emotionally.

A good fit with services in the community can enhance a patient's quality of life and enable them to live in the community successfully (Cohen, Gantt and Sainz, 1997). This can be difficult to achieve with this population, given the dual stigma of mental illness and sexual minority status that is so internalized for many. For example, a 58-year-old client who participated in the LGBT program for several years improved considerably. He decided to volunteer with an organization providing food to individuals with HIV. He found that the volunteers worked together as an intimate, close knit group, and he left, uncomfortably realizing that he was not yet ready to confront and share how in his 50s, he remained an unemployed college graduate as a consequence of chronic mental illness.

A male patient left the program when a gay, male therapist could not be assigned. A severely paranoid woman found an initial sense of "sympatico" in the program, but began attributing her delusional perceptions to staff and peers, and was lost to follow up after being rehospitalized. Another patient, who had felt something amiss despite work with a therapist of many years whom he described as supportive of his sexuality, eventually clarified his previous sense of incompleteness after referral to the support group, with its newfound social interaction with LGBT peers. Finally, to date, no one, to our knowledge, in the general client population has regressed or decompensated because of the inclusion and public availability of LGBT information in the clinic.

CONSUMER SATISFACTION SURVEY

Despite the best efforts of the program in its first few years, it was observed that attendance in the LGBT groups could be quite erratic. An effort was needed to clarify client needs and the overall impact of the then, four-year-old program.

In May 2000, a psychology graduate student, three LGBT patients, and the program director developed an anonymous "consumer satisfaction survey." This was distributed to LGBT clients attending the clinic over a two-week period. The survey consisted of 19 multiple choice and 6 open-ended questions. Twenty-two individuals responded to the survey. Results of the multiple-choice questions are listed in Table 1.

The largest group of clients in the program (63.6%) were gay men. It is unclear whether there is a lower demographic representation of gay women in this population, or if women are more reluctant to participate, or seek support elsewhere. Virtually all LGBT subjects (95.5%) felt "somewhat" to "very" comfortable in this mainstream clinic setting because of the LGBT program. Almost two-thirds (63.7%) were able to be more open, while 68.2% reported their mental health had improved because of the LGBT program "very much" or "somewhat." Seventy percent felt they received better treatment in the LGBT program than they had received elsewhere. Most (81.8%) found it beneficial to see culturally relevant information and materials displayed in the clinic.

More than four-fifths of the sample (81.8%) felt it was "very" to "somewhat" important to know their clinician was affiliated with the LGBT program. Almost all subjects were satisfied with their therapist (90%) and psychiatrist (95%). Most (85%) found staff to be sensitive to the needs of LGBT clients. About half (52.4%) regarded LGBT groups to be an integral part of their treatment. Of those not attending groups, 58.8% reported doing fine without the groups. The remainder felt the groups did not meet their needs. In this subset, comments included: already attending a group outside the clinic; uncertainty about the purpose of the group; not being comfortable with groups; finding individual sessions with the therapist and psychiatrist sufficient; and, one request for better facilitation of the groups.

The survey suggests that this population needs considerable time within the safe environment of the program setting. Over three-fourths of the sample (76.2%) reported no increase in involvement with LGBT community organizations or events since entering the program. Respondents were also more re-

TABLE 1. Consumer Satisfaction Survey

Survey Question					
1. How do you identify yourself?	Lesbian	Gay	Bisexual	Transgender	Other
N	3	14	1	3	1
%	13.6	63.6	4.5	13.6	4.5
2. How comfortable have you felt at Heights Hill knowing there is an LGBT program?	Very much so	Somewhat	A little	Not at all	Not sure
N	15	6	1	0	0
%	68.2	27.3	4.5	0	0
3. Have you been able to be more open about yourself because of the LGBT program?	Very much so	Somewhat	A little	Not at all	Not sure
N	10	4	3	3	2
%	45.5	18.2	13.6	13.6	9.1
4. Do you feel your mental health has improved because of the LGBT program?	Very much so	Somewhat	A little	Not at all	Not sure
N	9	6	5	1	1
%	40.9	27.3	22.7	4.5	4.5
5. How does Heights Hill compare with treatment you have received elsewhere?	Much better	Somewhat better	About the same	Not quite as good	Not as good at all
N	10	4	6	0	0
%	50	20	30	0	0
6. Do you feel that LGBT groups are an integral part of your treatment?	Very much so	Somewhat	A little	Not at all	Not sure
N	6	5	4	1	5
%	28.6	23.8	19.0	4.8	23.8
7. If not currently attending any LGBT groups, is it because you are doing fine without the group or because the groups do not meet your needs?	I'm doing fine without the group	The groups offered don't quite meet my needs	I am currently attending LGBT groups		
N	10	7	3		
%	50	35	15		
8. Does it make a difference to know that your mental health provider is affiliated with the LGBT program?	Very much so	Somewhat	A little	Not at all	Not sure
N	12	6	1	3	0
%	54.5	27.3	4.5	13.6	0

9. The Heights Hill Clinic has displayed posters, rainbow flags, and brochures about the LGBT program. Has it been beneficial to you to see such materials displayed?	Very much so	Somewhat	A little	Not at all	Not sure
N	11	7	3	0	1
%	50.0	31.8	13.6	0	4.5
10. What changes would you like to see in the LGBT program? (Subjects could choose all that apply)	Self-help groups	More social activities	Help finding volunteer positions in the LGBT community	Help finding employment in the LGBT community	A residence for the LGBT consumer
N	5	3	3	10	5
%	15.2	9.1	9.1	30.3	15.2
	Family therapy	Helping new LGBT consumers at Heights-Hill	Other		
N	1	2	4		
%	3.0	6.1	12.1		
11. Have you attended a LGBT group here in the past?	Yes	No			
N	9	13			
%	40.9	59.1			
12. Do you find it convenient or difficult to get to Heights Hill?	Very convenient	Convenient	Not a problem	Somewhat inconvenient	Pretty difficult
N	9	6	1	3	2
%	42.9	28.6	4.8	14.3	9.5
13. Are you satisfied with the services you are receiving from your therapist?	Very satisfied	Satisfied	Neutral	Somewhat dissatisfied	Very dissatisfied
N	11	7	1	1	0
%	55.0	35.0	5.0	5.0	0
14. Are you satisfied with the services you are receiving from your psychiatrist?	Very satisfied	Satisfied	Neutral	Somewhat dissatisfied	Very dissatisfied
N	12	7	1	0	0
%	60.0	35.0	5.0	0	0
15. Do you feel that the reception staff treats you courteously and in a professional manner?	Very satisfied	Satisfied	Neutral	Somewhat dissatisfied	Very dissatisfied
N	9	6	2	2	2
%	42.9	28.6	9.5	9.5	9.5

TABLE 1 (continued)

Survey Question					
16. Are Heights Hill staff sensitive to the needs of LGBT consumers?	Very much so	Somewhat	Neutral	Somewhat insensitive	Very insensitive
N	12	5	3	0	0
%	60.0	25.0	15.0	0	0
17. Since being in our program, have you become more involved in LGBT events or organizations in the community?	Definitely	Somewhat	Not really	No	
N	1	4	6	10	
%	4.8	19.0	28.6	47.6	
18. Would you like more support connecting with resources in the community?	Definitely	Probably	Maybe	Probably not	No
N	5	3	3	6	3
%	25.0	15.0	15.0	30.0	15.0
19. Would you recommend the LGBT program at Heights Hill to someone you know?	Definitely	Probably	Maybe	Probably not	No
N	12	6	2	1	0
%	57.1	28.6	9.5	4.8	0

luctant about getting help connecting with LGBT community resources: 45% would decline such help, but 40% were interested. Still, a fourth of the sample had participated in outside community activities, and another two-fifths indicated an interest.

The change most requested in programming (30%) was provision of help finding employment in the LGBT community. Self-help groups and an LGBT residence were the next most desired changes (15.2% each). More than four-fifths of respondents (85.7%) would recommend the program to others.

The consumer satisfaction survey resulted in efforts to enhance the groups and self-help opportunities, expand networking with other LGBT responsive agencies to fill in service gaps such as LGBT sensitive residence placements, obtain funding to create peer-related jobs, and develop an LGBT social club.

CONCLUSION

The LGBT Affirmative Program at South Beach Psychiatric Center began in response to a recognized absence of psychosocial services for LGBT individuals with major mental illness. Initial staff concerns were addressed, and the program is now viewed as a resource to the clinic and the community. The program provides opportunities for the destigmatization and positive reinforcement of sexual minority status in individuals with major psychiatric disorders who would, otherwise, have difficulty utilizing the limited resources available within the LGBT and psychiatric communities. It provides opportunities for socialization previously unavailable, and strives to engender a sense of community and heritage.

In working with the mentally ill, Goering and Stylianos (1988) describe the need for a "real" and "human" relationship to take place within a therapeutic environment. The particular normative standard set for this program, framed by sexual and gender variation, demonstrates that culturally focused mental health services for sexual minorities can nourish and grow fuller human beings despite years of alienation and isolation.

The consumer survey indicates that patients are highly satisfied with the program in general, but challenges remain. Psychiatric symptoms, drug abuse, and personality disorders can be substantial obstacles in managing any program, no matter how culturally appropriate. Job, residence, inpatient, and family resources are needed. And, existing program components require regular review. The program recently evaluated a client for intake who initially commented that the clinic looked no different from others where she had received treatment before. She implied that there was nothing that immediately spoke to her need for a sense of gay community here. This, we continue to learn how to better understand our clients' range of needs and develop ways to make them feel more comfortable.

Program development and change does not occur overnight. Nor does its impact. Only in the later years of the program have we seen a more cohesive sexual minority community emerge within the clinic, as social identities have differentiated and grown. There is a new supportive "family" here, and a palpable sense of confidence that has materialized among many of these clients. It developed in a setting reflective of their culture, but it is often visible in their new relationship to the dominant heterosexual culture. It started with "family members" like themselves, and grew to include "non-family members," such as staff and other clients sensitive enough and experienced enough to be trusted, and interested enough to visit, learn, and live within their cultural milieu.

REFERENCES

Aponte, J., Rivers, R. & Wohl, J., eds. (1995), *Psychological Interventions and Cultural Diversity.* Boston, MA: Allyn & Bacon.
Bayer, R. (1981), *Homosexuality and American Psychiatry: The Politics of Diagnosis.* New York: Basic Books.

Cabaj, R.P. & Stein, T.S., eds. (1996), *Textbook of Homosexuality and Mental Health*. Washington, DC: American Psychiatric Press.

Cohen, N., Gantt, A.B. & Sainz, A. (1997), Influences on fit between psychiatric patient's psychotherapy social needs and their hospital discharge plan. *Psychiatric Services*, 48:518-523.

Ford, C.S. & Beach, F.A. (1951), *Patterns of Sexual Behavior*. New York: Basic Books.

Goering, P.N. & Stylianos, S.K. (1988), Exploring the helping relationship between the schizophrenic client and rehabilitation therapists. *American J. Orthopsychiaty*, 58:271-280.

Gonsiorek, J. (1982), Organizational and staff problems in gay/lesbian mental health agencies. In: *Homosexuality & Psychotherapy*, ed. J. Gonsiorek. New York: The Haworth Press.

Graham, M. (1998), *Cultural Competency in Mental Health Systems*. National Mental Health Association Position Statement, June.

Hellman, R. (1996), Issues in the treatment of lesbians and gay men with chronic mental Illness. *Psychiatric Services*, 47:1093-1098.

Hooker, E. (1957), The adjustment of the male overt homosexual. *J. Projective Techniques*, 21:18-30.

Kinsey, A., Pomeroy, W. & Martin, C. (1948), *Sexual Behavior in the Human Male*. Philadelphia, PA: Saunders.

Kinsey, A., Pomeroy, W., Martin, C. & Gebhard, P. (1953), *Sexual Behavior in the Human Female*. Philadelphia, PA: Saunders.

Leigh, J.W. (1998), *Communicating for Cultural Competence*. Boston, MA: Allyn and Bacon.

Lesbian, Gay, Bisexual, Transgender Hygiene Issues Committee (1998), New York City Federation for Mental Health, Mental Retardation, and Alcoholism Services. Unpublished survey.

Lewes, K. (1988), *The Psychoanalytic Theory of Male Homosexuality*. New York: Simon and Schuster.

Marmor, J., ed. (1965), *Sexual Inversion: The Multiple Roots of Homosexuality*. New York: Basic Books.

McCarn, S. (1999), Meeting the mental health needs of gay, lesbian, bisexual, and transgender persons. *Cultural Diversity Series*. National Technical Assistance Center for State Mental Health Planning, 2, August.

National Mental Health Association (1999), Best (& Worst) Practices in Private Sector Managed Mental Healthcare. NMHA Website (*http://www.nmha.org/shcr/bestprac/cultcomp.cfm*), May.

Soreff, S., ed. (1996), *Handbook for the Treatment of the Seriously Mentally Ill*. Seattle: Hogrefe & Huber.

Szasz, T. (1974), *The Myth of Mental Illness*. New York: Harper and Row.

Providing Mental Health Services for LGBT Teens in a Community Adolescent Health Clinic

Daniel M. Medeiros, MD
Mavis Seehaus, CSW
Jennifer Elliott, CSW
Adam Melaney, CSW

SUMMARY. Providing mental health services in a public setting to adolescents who are lesbian, gay, bisexual, transgender and questioning (LGBTQ) can be difficult due to multiple potential barriers. This article describes the process of successful engagement of these adolescents into services at Mount Sinai's Adolescent Health Center (MSAHC), with emphasis on group treatment. MSAHC is one of the oldest adolescent focused centers in the country that integrates mental health services into primary care. Grant funding supports the center's mission to provide services to teens regardless of ability to pay. The screening process and mental health services available to these adolescents are described. Four

Daniel M. Medeiros is Assistant Professor in the Department of Psychiatry at St. Luke's Roosevelt Hospital, and Director of the Adolescent Alternative Day Program and the Comprehensive Addiction Program for Adolescents at St. Luke's Roosevelt Hospital in New York City.

Mavis Seehaus, Jennifer Elliott, and Adam Melaney are all CSW social workers at the Mount Sinai Adolescent Health Center, and are staff of the Social Work Department of Mount Sinai Hospital.

Address correspondence to: Daniel M. Medeiros (E-mail: dmedeiros@chpnet.org).

[Haworth co-indexing entry note]: "Providing Mental Health Services for LGBT Teens in a Community Adolescent Health Clinic." Medeiros, Daniel M. et al. Co-published simultaneously in *Journal of Gay & Lesbian Psychotherapy* (The Haworth Medical Press, an imprint of The Haworth Press, Inc.) Vol. 8, No. 3/4, 2004, pp. 83-95; and: *Handbook of LGBT Issues in Community Mental Health* (ed: Ronald E. Hellman, and Jack Drescher) The Haworth Medical Press, an imprint of The Haworth Press, Inc., 2004, pp. 83-95. Single or multiple copies of this article are available for a fee from The Haworth Document Delivery Service [1-800-HAWORTH, 9:00 a.m. - 5:00 p.m. (EST). E-mail address: docdelivery@haworthpress.com].

different adolescent LGBTQ groups are reviewed, including how the groups were created and the goals of the groups. Problems encountered in the group process are outlined, each of which needed to be resolved in order to maintain the success of the group. *[Article copies available for a fee from The Haworth Document Delivery Service: 1-800-HAWORTH. E-mail address: <docdelivery@haworthpress.com> Website: <http://www.HaworthPress. com> © 2004 by The Haworth Press, Inc. All rights reserved.]*

KEYWORDS. Adolescents, AIDS, bisexual youth, gay youth, group therapy, HIV, lesbian youth, mental health services, psychoeducation, public psychiatry, safer sex, support groups, transgender youth

In 2001, the Surgeon General, David Satcher, released a report on children's mental health services recommending that these services be made more readily available in primary care settings in order to improve access (Department of Health and Human Services, 2001). The Mount Sinai Adolescent Health Center (AHC) is one of the oldest adolescent focused centers in the country and has integrated mental health services into primary care since its inception over thirty years ago.

It has been estimated that only 20% of children and adolescents with mental illness receive services (Kestenbaum, 2000), which is likely due to lack of access and the stigma of attending a mental health clinic. Yet, it is also estimated that half of adolescent medical visits are due to psychosocial issues (Rappaport, 2001). In addition, it is likely that teens already feeling stigmatized–such as LGBT teens and HIV-positive teens–would be even less able to overcome the added stigma of attending a mental health clinic. The Adolescent Health Center normalizes the process of seeking mental health treatment by having it as an integral part of comprehensive services.

In New York State, adolescents are entitled to confidential reproductive and mental health care (Feierman, Lieberman and Chu, 1996), but in reality they may find it hard to obtain. Using parental insurance can generate bills and statements of benefits that come to the parents' attention and compromise the teen's confidentiality. This may be of particular concern for LGBT and HIV-positive teens. In addition, many adolescents in New York City are uninsured (Smith et al., 2000, McCormick et al., 2000). In order to provide services to those who are uninsured or unwilling to use their parents' insurance due to confidentiality risks, AHC has received funding through multiple grants to support the center's services.[1] These grants allow the center to provide services to teens regardless of ability to pay. AHC serves adolescents primarily from East Harlem and the South Bronx, but young people from all five boroughs attend the center.

AHC is an adolescent-focused environment that embraces diversity. The walls are outlined with multicolored handprints from staff and clients, including several rainbow colored hands. Among the various posters, which include pictures from the teen parenting program, and posters from drug abuse contests, there is one of a rainbow flag, and posters for both the girls and boys same sex groups which were each designed by the participants of these groups. Pamphlets on sexuality are readily available. The staff also reflect the diversity of the clients served.

All mental health services at AHC are provided through four teams. The primary care team, which also includes two social workers from our school-based clinics, provides mental health care immediately through our medical clinics when a medical provider refers a teen to one of our social workers. Most of the transgender teens who are in medical care and receive hormones are seen by this team. Other LGBT teens seen for medical treatment may also be referred. The health educators who provide HIV testing may also refer adolescents, especially if there are concerns regarding high-risk behaviors.

The Ryan White team also accepts immediate referrals, as above, for HIV-affected youth. When an adolescent has a positive HIV test, a Ryan White social worker is assigned, and this worker is part of the post-test counseling with the health educator. The Ryan White social worker facilitates the required services that the newly diagnosed teen needs. In addition, HIV-positive adolescents in medical service elsewhere are often referred to AHC because of the comprehensive, adolescent-focused mental health services, including two successful HIV-positive support groups for youth. Of the fifty positive teens currently in service, half are young males who contracted HIV through same sex encounters. HIV-affected adolescents are also referred through our mental health intake process, which is similar to the referrals for our other two mental health teams.

Adolescent clients can be referred directly for mental health services through a telephone intake process that schedules new clients for the two mental health teams. Referrals come from schools throughout the city, parents, social service agencies, and through the young people themselves, usually through word of mouth. During the first scheduled evaluation the client fills out the Adquest (Adolescent Questionnaire), which was developed at AHC in order to obtain the teen's view of their concerns and the issues they are interested in talking about. On the Adquest (Peake, 2000) there is one question on sexual orientation as follows:

How would you describe yourself? (Check any below)
Straight (Heterosexual)___   Bisexual___
Gay___   Transgender___
Lesbian___   Not Sure___

Of the 487 surveys processed, we have recorded the following results:

> Ninety-five percent of the boys identified as being heterosexual, while 85% of the girls did. Seventy-four percent of white teens identified as being straight. Eighty-nine percent of African Americans and 91% of Latinos and West Indian/Caribbean identified as being straight. These surveys are reflective of the two mental health teams and do not include the LGBT teens or other youth seen in primary care or the HIV-positive adolescents involved in Ryan White.

All of AHC's mental health services are available to all AHC clients, which include individual, family and group therapy, psychological testing, psychiatric evaluation, and psychiatric medication management. In addition, some of the clients may participate in the center's vocational mentorship program, summer youth employment program, or our peer education program. Approximately fifty percent of the clients have serious impairment of functioning, indicated by a Global Assessment of Functioning (GAF) of 50 or lower. All the transgender youth and the HIV-positive youth receive a baseline psychiatric evaluation as part of their assessment package. Because group affiliation is a strong component of adolescent development and because very little has been written about group treatment in this population, this paper discusses the history of four adolescent LGBT focused groups developed at AHC. These are the Lesbian, Bisexual and Questioning[2] Girls Group, the Gay, Bisexual and Questioning Boys Group, the Transgender Tea Party, and the HIV-Positive Support Group for Gay and Bisexual Males.

THE LESBIAN, BISEXUAL AND QUESTIONING GIRLS GROUP

The Lesbian, Bisexual and Questioning Girls Group was started at the Adolescent Health Center because the girls requested it. Girls coming to the mental health program or the primary care clinic requested a group with girls like themselves, where they could openly discuss dating and sex, among other issues, without feeling "different." In the couple of years preceding the start of the group, AHC staff became increasingly aware that gay and lesbian youth are less likely to seek health care than heterosexual teens, and they are often reluctant to disclose for fear of being judged. Staff became more conscious of asking questions in a non-heterosexist manner and displayed materials designed for gay and lesbian youth, thereby demonstrating their willingness to be supportive. This environment facilitated the girls being able to ask for what they wanted and needed.

The purpose of the group was several-fold. A major developmental task of gay, lesbian and bisexual youth is adjustment to a socially stigmatized sexual role and identity. The group was intended to facilitate support around these issues and encourage feelings of pride in their identities. These issues arose almost immediately, as the girls discussed their experiences of discrimination and gay bashing but also their determination to feel good about themselves. The group also gave the girls an opportunity to explore decisions regarding dating and sex in a safe environment. To improve their knowledge and risk-reducing skills in this area, a health educator, specializing in sexual health, visited the group on a regular basis to teach and answer questions. The group also focused on decision-making related to coming out to family and others. Questioning youth learned from peers that they were fine whether they ultimately felt they were gay, bisexual or straight and were relieved in not being told they were "just going through a phase." The group gave some of its members an opportunity to meet other lesbian, bisexual and questioning girls for the first time, addressing feelings of isolation, not uncommon to gay people during their teen years. Group members spent much time discussing issues common to all teenagers. Knowing they would not be judged for their identity issues facilitated their comfort and openness.

The group met for several years with the same four to six core group members, as other members came and went. One of the group's first tasks was to name the group. After much discussion, it was called "US," which stood for "United Sexualities," designed to welcome all. Initially, the group leaders led some icebreaker exercises but it quickly became clear that the girls would rather have less structure and raise issues themselves. The group met during the school year and broke for the summer every year. During the last meeting before the summer break, the group would do an activity, such as seeing a gay-themed movie or visiting a gay bookstore.

One of the challenges of the group was how to handle dating between group members. Initially the leader had a "no dating" rule due to concerns that relationship conflicts would not be openly addressed in the group and eventually members would drop out of the group. However, this rule was found to be counterproductive, as members began to date secretly. The leader was not informed and could not address the resulting conflict appropriately, which did result in some drop out. Once this rule was suspended, there has been more overt flirtation, but this is now more easily addressed and negotiated in the group.

Most of the girls were also in individual therapy, but some attended group only, and were not interested in individual treatment. However, when clients revealed risk behaviors that would benefit from a more intensive treatment, such as individual therapy, it was difficult to convince them of the potential advantage. Generally, these clients would then be seen by the group leader instead of being referred to another therapist for individual therapy.

Over time, the girls became supports to one another outside the group. They met on school holidays, attended each other's proms and visited agencies for gay youth together. When several of the girls began college, the group went on a hiatus. But, due to patient interest, it has recently been reformed with new membership.

GAY, BISEXUAL AND QUESTIONING BOYS GROUP

The gay, bisexual and questioning boys group developed as a result of providing individual and group psychotherapy to HIV-positive adolescents in the Ryan White program. The HIV-positive gay and bisexual patients stated that therapy helped them not only to address their medical issues, but also to come to terms with their sexual orientation and explore their sexuality in a safe and responsible manner. They felt that if they could process sexual identity issues before, or early on in their sexual experimentation, they might avoid HIV infection.

AHC staff began to identify HIV-negative gay, bisexual and questioning young men in their caseloads and referred these patients to be assessed for group. These young men were primarily Latino and African American from Harlem and Spanish Harlem and ranged in age from 16-22. Two months later, the Gay, Bisexual and Questioning Boys Group was born. The original facilitators were both openly gay men. It became clear to the facilitators that the group would have three main goals: to allow the young men to process, accept and integrate their feelings of same-sex attraction in an affirming and nurturing environment, to help them define and follow through with safer sex practices (all members had already engaged in sexual activity), and to develop "healthy" dating/relationship dynamics.

Most of the adolescents reported having sex in cruising areas in parks, clubs/backrooms, or meeting older men on the Internet and going over to their homes for sex. Sexual activity was disconnected from the rest of their lives as a way to distance and manage the overwhelming guilt and shame. These teens tended to avoid, inhibit, and cut off their same-sex attraction during most of the day, then resort to sexual exploration in situations and environments that were cut-off and disconnected from their "real life." The youth had quick, furtive sexual experiences that were fulfilling their sexual need in the moment, but the sexual experience occurred in a dissociated state, mired in guilt and shame.

It is in this state that the adolescents found themselves denying the necessity for using condoms and practicing safer sex that would lower the risk of HIV infection. Creating the group space for the gay, bisexual and questioning young men to share their thoughts and feelings with supportive peers and facilitators who normalized their internal experiences allowed the participants to accept their same-sex attractions and begin to create a self-defined identity as a gay or bisexual man. As comfort with sexual identity solidified in the group, members more fully self-identified in the world at large. As these young men began feeling increasingly comfortable identifying as gay or bisexual men, group conversations moved from a preoccupation with sexual fantasies and sexual encounters to a focus on dating, relationships, and love with other men. During this period, participants reported being less fulfilled by furtive encounters in the parks and other anonymous sex situations.

The group spent a great deal of time struggling with the question of sex versus relationship. Eventually, the group came to a consensus that one did not have to choose between the two but could have both. As the members began to lose interest in anonymous sex in risky environments, they ventured into meeting age-appropriate partners in more suitable environments. Participants expressed anger and frustration that their straight peers were able to meet potential dates almost anywhere, but they, as gay and bisexual young men, were forced to go to gay community centers/agencies/functions/clubs to meet other young men. The group began to focus on issues of meeting and dating men their own age. Most participants found it very challenging to relate in a nonsexual manner and to get to know the person before having sex. The group compared "normal sexual development" of their straight peers to their own experiences of meeting men just for sex and recognized the dangers and risks the group members had been taking. The group began to value dating as a preferred alternative to having a one-night stand, and group members began to see the possibility that they could lead a "normal life" just like straight adolescents; they could meet other males their age, date, fall in love, and have a family.

Throughout the group sessions, facilitators provided psychoeducation regarding HIV. Initially, the participants were reticent to discuss their thoughts and feelings about HIV, and simply listened to the facilitators present information. Most of the participants had a poor level of knowledge about HIV and its transmission. During the first couple of months, participants stated their belief that because they did not self identify as "gay," they were not at risk. They also believed that because they had sex with married men in parks and other such environments, the men they had sex with could not have HIV, since they were not "gay" either. Others felt that as long as they were not anally penetrated, there was no real risk for HIV infection. Many members would smoke marijuana or drink alcohol before looking for sex, to help them cope with shame and guilt evoked by their same-sex attraction. Because of these factors, several of the youth had placed themselves at serious risk for HIV infection.

The facilitators provided psychoeducation regarding the basic knowledge of HIV transmission, reproduction, and treatment. The participants were surprised by some of the information and experienced a more realistic under-standing of the level of risk of their sexual practices. The facilitators spent two full sessions focusing on safer sex practices and eroticizing safer sex. At this point in the group process, members were very verbal and articulate about their sexual experiences and were able to actively absorb the information and understand that they could have sex that would be both fulfilling, and signifi-cantly decrease their exposure to HIV infection, by using, for example, con-doms.

Eight months into the group, one of the members asked the group leaders to join him in his individual session during which he told them that he had just re-ceived a positive test for HIV that day. After revealing this, he dropped out of the group. His abrupt departure did not allow other group members to process the termination of his treatment with him. Group members expressed strong feelings of betrayal and abandonment by this member, which the leaders ex-plored in depth. However, because the leaders were entrusted with the confi-dential information of the member's HIV status, they were also angry regarding some of the group members reactions. In group supervision, group leaders worked through feelings of helplessness and feelings that they had clinically failed this client and the group. In supervision, the group leaders were able to explore additional options to better handle this type of situation in the future.

Three years later, the Gay, Bisexual and Questioning Boys Group contin-ues to provide an opportunity for young men to discuss their same-sex attrac-tions and explorations, while minimizing their risk for HIV infection. Although the group facilitators and the patients who make up the group have changed, the commitment to provide a safe space for these young men to discuss their same-sex feelings and behaviors continues.

TRANSGENDER TEA PARTY

Several male-to-female (MTF) transgender adolescents have been fol-lowed at the Adolescent Health Center for feminizing hormone treatment and counseling. These young people, having had experiences of rejection and abuse related to their transgender identities, took much time to develop trust in their therapist and were initially apprehensive to meet one another. Feeling it would be beneficial for the adolescents to meet, the therapist and physician be-gan to schedule these patients the same afternoon so they could get to know one another informally. For some time, these patients were in different stages of transitioning from a more masculine to a more feminine appearance. Even-tually they were passing as females in their daily environments and all were exploring and struggling with the issue of disclosure, particularly in dating sit-uations. To facilitate discussion, support, safe decision-making regarding disclosure, and to gauge interest in future group activities, a tea party was planned.

The transgender patients were reluctant to attend support or therapy groups. Part of this resistance was their desire "to pass" and not identify as transgender. However, in time, they decided they were willing to come to a tea party to get together with other transgender youth. The participants were permitted to choose snacks and spent time together planning the menu. At the party, they initially bonded over topics such as favorite music and stores, but then discussed school, their neighborhoods and experiences with hormones. They were aware their therapist wanted to facilitate a discussion of disclosure, a very charged subject for them, and they began to ask, in a general way, about each other's views on this. When the group ended, they requested a monthly gathering and decided dating would be their next topic.

HIV-POSITIVE SUPPORT GROUP
FOR GAY AND BISEXUAL MALES

As the clinic began to provide services for more and more HIV-positive gay and bisexual males, it became apparent that they could benefit from a group that would address issues specific to their sexuality. Contact with social workers from other agencies working with HIV-positive adolescents also indicated that there was a need for such a group in the broader community, and the group leaders decided the group should include youth referred by outside medical and mental health programs. The group began with the purpose of allowing the young men an opportunity for mutual support around health and psychosocial issues, as well as providing psychosocial education about sex, HIV, STDs, and medications.

Potential members are referred to the group by their therapists or doctors and screened by one or both of the facilitators before they are able to join. Confidentiality has been an important concern during the screening, as the young men often fear that other members will disclose their HIV status in mutual social arenas. This concern is addressed during the initial group screening and in the group whenever a new member joins. Once the young men realize they each have the same fears, they have more trust in their privacy being maintained. All members have agreed that the most important topics to discuss include medications and adherence, dating, sex, disclosure (to friends, family and especially partners), and support from family regarding HIV status, sexuality, and establishing independence. The length of time since members were first diagnosed varies. This serves to further enhance support of one another, particularly for those recently diagnosed. During the screening, and in initial group encounters, facilitators reiterate the importance of a "no dating" rule between members, as a reminder that the group is not meant to be a dating service, but rather a place for support and discussion.

Membership in the group has fluctuated, with members' busy schedules causing the majority of problems in attendance. Each member has voiced his feeling of connection to the group, and most of them have spent time socially outside of group sessions. Facilitators allow the members to decide what will be discussed each week, but regularly question them about their attendance to medical appointments, status of their blood counts and adherence to medications. Almost every session involves a lengthy discussion of dating and new partners, and whether HIV status has been disclosed. Members have been very open about this and have repeatedly helped each other make decisions about how and when to disclose, and how to negotiate protected sex with partners who do not know their status. The facilitators have been impressed with the young men's honesty and openness with each other, regardless of the more taboo subjects like anonymous sex, prostitution and unprotected sex. Group members generally agree that this is one of the few places where they are able to even voice their thoughts and feelings about such issues.

The group leaders had to actively set appropriate boundaries in order to maintain the safety of the group. For example, at one point a member became involved in an on-line video pornography business and several sessions were spent exploring the pros and cons of such involvement. When it became clear that this member was being paid extra money to refer other young men, and that he had taken another group member to sign up, the leaders became quite concerned. In the group leaders' supervision, it was decided to address this member individually. The group member was told the clinic would not allow recruitment and that this needed to be addressed in the group. Individual therapists of the group members were also informed, in order to allow the issue to be addressed individually with each member. This disruptive group member missed several groups after this limit was set, but the rest of the group was able to process what had happened and discuss at length why this caused concern for the group leaders and the clinic as a whole. Leaders emphasized the importance of members feeling safe to bring up any issues for discussion, without the risk of coercion or manipulation by staff or other members of the group.

The HIV-Positive Support Group for Gay and Bisexual Males has highlighted for the AHC staff the myriad issues that affect these young men daily, and how their sexuality and HIV status are intertwined. It serves as an important forum for them to discuss very difficult topics in a supportive and understanding environment, without fear of judgment. Each member has been able to hear how others are going through the same difficulties and thus find reassurance that they are not alone. It is hoped that with this support, the young men will be able to continue to learn the skills necessary for developing a sense of self-worth and pride in their sexual identities, and that this will also encourage them to maintain their health and safety.

CONCLUSION

There are many potential barriers that can prevent LGBT and HIV-positive teens from receiving mental health care. New York State law requires that adolescents be able to receive confidential sexuality and mental health treatment. Grant funding allows these youth to be seen without fear of having confidentiality broken due to billing issues, and allows for comprehensive visits during which a teen can see a medical provider, health educator, nutritionist, social worker and psychiatrist all on the same day. Having comprehensive services in one location decreases the stigma of seeking another place for mental health services and provides for better integration of services for complex issues such as HIV.

An adolescent focused center helps young people feel more assured that their care is confidential, and sexuality issues and mental health issues can be addressed more openly as part of good care. Having a staff and physical environment that is reflective of the population being served, and that is warm and welcoming, encourages teens to bring up sensitive issues, as does not assuming a heterosexist bias when asking questions. It is also important to have a "critical mass" so that LGBT adolescents do not feel that they are "the only one." Groups are a very powerful way of helping LGBT young people support each other.

Public funding provides the flexibility to run groups whenever needed, for as long as needed, without concern for limitations on the number of authorized visits. It is critical for programs to address as many of these barriers as possible in order to successfully address the unmet needs of this underserved population.

NOTES

1. Grants include a New York State (NYS) Department of Health (DOH) family planning grant, a NYS Office of Alcoholism and Substance Abuse Services (OASAS) substance prevention grant, a NYS DOH violence prevention and treatment grant, federal Ryan White funding for HIV infected/affected youth which is administered through state and city agencies, and a recent federal Substance Abuse and Mental Health Services Administration (SAMHSA) grant for trauma treatment.
2. The term "questioning" has recently appeared in the literature (DeVries, 1998, Morrison and L'Heureux, 2001, Russell and Osher, 2001) but no source has been found which defines the term, and this term is likely being used in different ways. An excel-

lent book, *Lesbian & Gay Youth, Care & Counseling* (Ryan and Futterman, 1998), sheds some light on what the term encompasses:

> Although the majority of adolescents are aware of their sexual feelings and some acknowledge sexual orientation during early adolescence, many do not consolidate sexual identity until their early 20s. Thus, adolescence for many lesbian and gay youth is characterized by indecision, uncertainty, and vacillation between heterosexual, bisexual or homosexual labels. (p. 29)
>
> When youth are questioning or confused about sexual identity, vulnerability is increased, and support is particularly important. (p. 100)
>
> In four surveys of young males, the prevalence of same-sex activity to orgasm ranged from 17-37%, however, the percentage who later self-identify as gay is much lower. Moreover, many adolescents who later identify as lesbian or gay may self-label as bisexual when they are younger. In a survey of lesbian and gay youth, ages 14-21, for example, more than half had previously identified as bisexual. (p. 106)

In addition, substantial variation exists across racial and ethnic groups concerning the social acceptability of exact orientations and identities (Dean et al., 2000), and for some in the African American community, "taking on a gay identity means giving up an African American identity" (Stokes and Peterson, 1998). The Centers for Disease Control and Prevention (CDC) has reported that as many as 24% of homosexually active African American men with HIV identified themselves as heterosexual, as well as 15% of Latino men (CDC, 2000). Given that the population at AHC consists of multicultural youth who may not have a solid sexual identity or may resist being labeled gay, lesbian or bisexual, offering the term "questioning" may be more acceptable to these adolescents and make it more likely that they would seek out the group to explore their sexual feelings.

REFERENCES

Centers for Disease Control and Prevention (2000), HIV/AIDS among racial/ethnic minority men who have sex with men–United States, 1989-1998. *MMWR*, 49:1.
Dean, L., Meyer, I., Robinson, K., Sell, R., Sember, R., Silenzio, V., Bowen, D., Bradford, J., Rothblum, E., Scout, M., White, J., Dunn, P., Lawrence, A., Wolfe, D. & Xavier, J. (2000), Lesbian, gay, bisexual, and transgender health: Findings and concerns. *J. Gay & Lesbian Medical Association*. 4:101-151.
Department of Health and Human Services (2001), *Report of the Surgeon General's Conference on Children's Mental Health: A National Action Agenda*. Department of Human Services Website (*http: //surgeongeneral.gov/cmh/childreport.htm*).
De Vries, G. (1998), Issues affecting gay, lesbian, bisexual, transgender, and questioning youth. *Los Angeles: Family and Conciliation Courts Review*, 36:417-419.
Feierman, J., Lieberman, D. & Chu, Y. (1996), *Teenagers Health Care & the Law: A Guide to the Law on Minors' Rights in New York*. New York, NY: Civil Liberties Union Reproductive Rights Project.

Kestenbaum, C. (2000), How shall we treat the children in the 21st century. *J. American Academy Child & Adolescent Psychiatry*, 39:1-10.

McCormick, M., Kass, B., Elixhauser, A., Thompson, J. & Simpson, L. (2000), Annual report on access to and utilization of health care for children and youth in the United States–1999. *Pediatrics*, 105:219-230.

Morrison, L. & L'Heureux, J. (2001). Suicide and gay/lesbian/bisexual youth: Implications for clinicians. *J. Adolescence*, 24:39-49.

Peake, K. (2000), *Practice-Based Research and the Development of the Reflective Organization*. New York: City University of New York, unpublished dissertation.

Rappaport, N. (2001), Psychiatric consultation to school-based health centers: Lessons learned in an emerging field. *J. American Academy Child & Adolescent Psychiatry*, 40: 1473-1475.

Russell, S. & Osher, J. (2001), *LGBTQ Youth Are at Risk in U.S. School Environment*. New York: SIECUS Report.

Ryan, C. & Futterman, D. (1998). *Lesbian & Gay Youth: Care & Counseling*. New York: Columbia University Press.

Smith, L., Wise, P., Chavkin, W., Romero, D. & Zuckerman, B. (2000), Implications of welfare reform for child health: Emerging challenges for clinical practice and policy. *Pediatrics*, 106:1117-1125.

Stokes, J. & Peterson, J. (1998), Homophobia, self-esteem and risk for HIV among African American men who have sex with men. *AIDS Education & Prevention*, 10: 278-292.

The Community Health Project

Daniel Garza, MD

SUMMARY. The onset of the AIDS crisis led to a coalition of various
community agencies and medical professional volunteers to form the
Community Health Project (CHP) in the Chelsea area of New York City.
The lesbian, gay, bisexual and transgender (LGBT) individuals that fre-
quented this primary care facility led to its further development into the
Michael Callen-Audre Lorde Community Health Center. As the first,
and still the largest, fully licensed health care agency of its kind,
Callen-Lorde seeks to provide primary care to individuals regardless of
their ability to pay. Mental health services have also grown within the
organization and are a key component of the specialized divisions providing care. Services include counseling for HIV-related issues, transgender biopsychosocial assessments, and the incorporation of psychiatry
into the care provided in the adolescent and young adult division of the
facility. The persisting marginalization of many in the LGBT community underscores the need for further efforts to explore the provision of
services in the public health arena for this population. *[Article copies available for a fee from The Haworth Document Delivery Service: 1-800-HAWORTH.
E-mail address: <docdelivery@haworthpress.com> Website: <http://www.
HaworthPress.com> © 2004 by The Haworth Press, Inc. All rights reserved.]*

Daniel Garza is Assistant Clinical Professor of Psychiatry at Mt. Sinai Medical
Center, and is the Consulting Psychiatrist for the Health Outreach to Teens Program of
the Michael Callen-Audre Lorde Community Health Center.

Address correspondence to: Dr. Daniel Garza, AOT Program, Room C11-11,
Elmhurst Hospital, 79-01 Broadway, Elmhurst, NY 11373.

[Haworth co-indexing entry note]: "The Community Health Project." Garza, Daniel. Co-published simul-
taneously in *Journal of Gay & Lesbian Psychotherapy* (The Haworth Medical Press, an imprint of The
Haworth Press, Inc.) Vol. 8, No. 3/4, 2004, pp. 97-105; and: *Handbook of LGBT Issues in Community Mental
Health* (ed: Ronald E. Hellman, and Jack Drescher) The Haworth Medical Press, an imprint of The Haworth
Press, Inc., 2004, pp. 97-105. Single or multiple copies of this article are available for a fee from The Haworth
Document Delivery Service [1-800-HAWORTH, 9:00 a.m. - 5:00 p.m. (EST). E-mail address: docdelivery@
haworthpress.com].

http://www.haworthpress.com/web/JGLP
Digital Object Identifer: 10.1300/J236v08n03_07

KEYWORDS. AIDS, bisexual, Michael Callen, Community Health Project, gay, gay youth, HIV, homosexuality, lesbian, Audre Lorde, mental health services, primary care, queer, transgender

Over the West 18th Street entrance of the Callen-Lorde Community Health Center (CLCHC) in Manhattan is a large aluminum canopy that swoops out from a facade of frosted glass, interrupted by a metal grid of grassy green. Once inside the Center, it is clear that this is not the same clinic that once struggled to serve its lesbian, gay, bisexual and transgender (LGBT) population. In 2003, its problems are those of any other health care facility operating in New York City: Medicaid, Medicare, third party payers, grants and affiliation contracts are what will determine the future of a facility such as CLCHC. However, twenty years ago the clinic was known as the Community Health Project (CHP), and 1983 was a very different era for such a place.

If one was lucky enough to have good health insurance in the 1970s, there was no guarantee that one's primary care facility provider would be "gay friendly." The Community Health Project, or CHP, was founded from the merger of two distinct agencies, the St. Mark's Community Clinic and The Gay Men's Health Project (not to be confused with today's Gay Men's Health Crisis). St Mark's Community Clinic provided counseling, crisis management and evaluations, but was not providing health care per se. Gay Men's Health Project provided on-site screening and referrals for those testing positive for sexually transmitted diseases. When both facilities joined forces, they provided a novel, grass roots level of care for the LGBT community. Many of those who accessed episodic care at CHP found, for the first time, health care that was non-judgmental, accessible, inexpensive and, more than anything else, safe for LGBT individuals.[1]

Originally, the merger created a facility that was largely staffed by volunteers, most of whom were gay and lesbian themselves. They created CHP in a setting partly occupied by a homeless shelter program. A space was renovated, again by volunteers, but CHP would eventually be situated in the Gay and Lesbian Community Center in New York's Greenwich Village.

It was a time when many individuals flocked to the West Village, not only for entertainment and a sense of community, but for their primary health care as well. From its inception, CHP offered health care to the community, regardless of an individual's ability to pay. The clinic operated on four separate nights, or Clinic groups, per week, and various individuals who worked there provided care after their day jobs. Supervision was minimal, but the clinic began to build on the experience and commitment of those volunteers, as well as developing creative approaches to meeting the needs of the community they served.

Of course, no discussion of health care could exclude the looming specter of HIV and AIDS. The development of institutions working with gay populations at this time was not just influenced by HIV–it molded them completely. As HIV permeated the gay community, many found themselves increasingly ostracized from mainstream venues of medical care (Shilts, 1987). Whatever shame might have existed for gay people in the past was now amplified by the onset of AIDS. The delivery of mental health care, within a total environment of LGBT health care delivery, was thus solidified by AIDS and its effects. Supportive counseling was an obvious focus in this scenario, as was crisis counseling, bereavement work, and family therapy. HIV spurred many gay people to seek help for mood disorders and cognitive deficits. The development of widespread and reliable HIV testing in the mid-80s led to a greater demand for counseling services. A positive test result was among the most foreboding of medical diagnoses, and psychological evaluation and support became a crucial component of treatment.

AIDS-related charitable organizations, governmental support of efforts to fight HIV, diagnostic and treatment facilities, and the mental health response to the disease all became increasingly linked. A biopsychosocial approach to HIV illness has since been the model for successful care.

From the second floor of the Lesbian and Gay Community Services Center, thousands of patients received health care, HIV-related and otherwise. By 1997, its fifteenth year at the Center, a staggering 20,000 patient-visits per year were being handled in a 2,500-square-foot space, seemingly confirming the paucity of alternative options for many LGBT individuals. Then, in 1997, to help address the growing demand, CHP moved into a $3.5 million center, which opened in an abandoned six-story warehouse in Chelsea, on 18th Street near Ninth Avenue. Renamed the Callen-Lorde Community Health Center (CLCHC),[2] it began to approach health care for the gay and lesbian community in the most comprehensive way possible. Callen-Lorde became the first LGBT agency in the United States designated as a Federally Qualified Health Center under Section 330(e) of the Public Health Service Act. The nearly ten-fold increase in physical area allowed for a more reasonable allocation of space, and the diversification and further development of many divisions within CHP, such as HIV treatment, Transgender Services, Senior Health Services and Lesbian Health Services. Now serving over 15,000 registered patients since its inception, it is the largest health center in the United States targeting the LGBT community.[3]

HEALTH OUTREACH TO TEENS (HOTT)

Over time, many innovative programs developed within the organization. One worth mentioning is the Health Outreach to Teens (HOTT) Program. A model agency that provides essentially free primary care to LGBT and questioning youth, ages 13-24, HOTT also seeks out homeless street youth, squatter populations and young people housed in social service and foster care housing agencies. Interestingly, a significant number of heterosexual clients are drawn to the program due to its non-judgmental, youth-oriented and confidential approach to the sexual and health care issues associated with adolescent and young adult development. Both gay and straight youth from the Tri-State area are seen waiting together for their appointments in the same physical space. The HOTT program is the only facility of its kind.

HOTT was initially situated within the CHP area, but many youth began to express a desire for a separate space away from the older, fully adult clientele seeking services. Many sought the safety of any locale where they felt they could be themselves and among their peers. The need to be around other queer youth was critical for many who traveled to the Village, out of a sense of isolation and discrimination in their own neighborhoods, schools and families. Still other youth were living on the streets of lower Manhattan, and had few places to seek refuge where they did not have to fear exploitation.

In the old space, CHP took all comers. This often resulted in gay white men taking care of gay white men, and a homeless teenager of color living on the streets might perceive the communal waiting room as less than hospitable. Furthermore, this younger population had less need for an HIV clinic then a sanctuary where they could be openly queer. The new facility on West 18th Street was a boon for these youth. Inhabiting the entire second floor of CLCHC, the HOTT program created its own entrance that youth can access directly from the lobby. They can wait for appointments in a youth-oriented atmosphere that is bright and well lit, and which provides videos, snacks and health educational materials that are aimed directly at them. Street youth can access the clothing bank and a shower provided within HOTT. Primary care and HIV pre- and post-test counseling are provided free of charge.

Transgender health care for youth is another maverick aspect of health care at HOTT. Few populations in today's society are more marginalized and discriminated against than transgender youth. Despite an increasingly well-informed medical establishment regarding gay and lesbian health care issues, to young persons questioning or rejecting their gender of birth, even health care in New York City can seem rejecting. A long-standing project of the clinic is its transgender hormonal therapy protocol. Developed after years of effort to meet the needs of individuals of transgender experience, hormonal therapy is offered in a multidisciplinary environment encompassing medical, mental health and social service care.

After a screening and evaluation that may last many months, young adults may qualify to receive hormonal therapy to assist in gender reassignment. The request for assistance with gender reassignment is, in fact, an opportunity for many psychosocial problems to be disclosed and addressed. A psychiatric screening is required, and may uncover trauma or mood-related symptoms that become a focus of treatment and additional support.

CLCHC utilizes a harm-reduction approach, so that youths who secure hormones on the street, or do not have adequate medical supervision can, nevertheless, access preventive care, such as regular lab tests, to ensure the safest possible use of hormones. In this way, HOTT provides a non-exploitative option for at-risk youth who are unable and unlikely to establish a more responsible health care connection elsewhere.

To ensure a comprehensive approach to primary health care and education, the HOTT program was able to secure funding through a grant from the Community Trust to provide on-sight psychiatric consultation and supervision. As part of the primary care team, the HOTT psychiatrist can assist in providing evaluation and treatment within the clinic. Given the age cohort of patients seeking assistance at the HOTT program, some may present with the first symptoms of a severe and persistent mental illness. This makes the presence of an in-house psychiatrist extremely convenient; many of these initial decompensations can be handled within the facility. More severe presentations are referred to inpatient or outpatient psychiatric facilities, which either stabilize and maintain the patients, or supplement the medical and psychiatric care provided by HOTT.

A PSYCHIATRIC PRESENCE

Psychiatric care at Callen-Lorde was initially provided through a unique relationship with Bellevue Hospital Center's Department of Psychiatry. Bellevue rented space from Callen-Lorde, yet clients seen within this satellite division of Bellevue were not technically receiving mental health services through CLCHC. Nevertheless, many would avail themselves of the queer friendly primary care services situated on other floors of the building. The relationship between Bellevue and CLCHC dissolved in 1998 when Bellevue closed their division in the building. Subsequently, no psychiatric services were accessible for the general adult clients of CLCHC, though psychiatric services were just being introduced to youth accessing the HOTT program.

Mental health services to adults within CHP, and initially at CLCHC, were provided by social workers through a consultation-liaison model that supported primary care providers. Psychiatry became available in the facility again in 2000 through an arrangement with Columbia University's Public Psychiatry fellowship program. The psychiatry fellows divide their time between lectures and supervision at the New York State Psychiatric Institute, and a work site in the public sector of their choosing.[4]

Psychiatry and other mental health services have always been in high demand at CLCHC. However, the psychiatrists' limited hours at the facility led to a need to develop a model of care provision that allowed maximum accessibility for clients without overwhelming their doctor's schedules. A framework was developed in which clients were referred for evaluations from in-house sources. Most of these individuals are diagnosed with anxiety and depressive disorders. After one or two visits, a recommendation is made. No further psychiatric management may be needed, but further stabilization is offered for crisis situations. Clients requiring more extensive management are referred to mental health providers outside Callen-Lorde. These have included gay-friendly agencies such as Federation Employment Guidance Services (FEGS), St. Vincent's Hospital, Greenwich House and Bellevue Hospital.

Yet, even these resources have limited accommodations because many CLCHC clients have financial limitations that require payment through sliding scales to receive care.[5] Diagnoses of severe or persistent mental illness can overwhelm the available resources offered by mental health providers in a primary care setting, and there is a persisting need to establish a mental health clinic as an equal partner with primary care.

LESBIAN HEALTH SERVICES DIVISION

During the early days of CHP, a lesbian presence in an environment initially designed to address the STD needs of white gay men was not an easy adjustment.[6] Issues of parenting and medical-legal liaison, domestic violence, and substance abuse were all crystallizing as areas needing attention in the lesbian community. Obviously, the mental health ramifications of a group all but invisible, until recently, from the general medical community and its research, could only be inferred. In 1999, the Institute of Medicine, a division of the National Academy of Science, issued a report identifying the need for studies that would clarify conditions for which the lesbian population would be susceptible. This came as a result of findings suggesting that many lesbians avoid addressing their primary care needs due to hostility in the medical community regarding their sexuality, or due to their discomfort discussing personal or other sexual matters with their doctors. Many lesbians simply ignored preventative health care. Though a lesbian health group began to develop in the days of CHP, in 1999 a more definitive coalescence of women providing care for other women began at CLCHC. Now addressing the needs of uninsured and under insured women, the Lesbian Health Services Division at CLCHC serves yet another clientele that may have future implications for additional service provision within psychiatry.

FUTURE HURDLES

According to Jay Laudato, CLCHC's Executive Director, mental health services would be all but absent were it not for funding from AIDS-related organizations. Though much mental health care is reimbursed or otherwise paid for by third-party payers, Medicaid, or Medicare, such treatment often needs to be intimately connected with the provision of healthcare for medical diagnoses. A stand-alone mental health clinic providing services for gays and lesbians has never drawn the necessary attention or money to become a viable entity. In today's fiscal climate, such a facility would be impossible to start without an overarching agency such as Callen-Lorde. Treatment groups for both HIV positive and negative men who have sex with men, long-term HIV survivors' groups, and transgender counseling and education are among the areas in which CLCHC strives to remain in the forefront of mental health care.

Yet much is still lacking in mental health service provision to the LGBT community. For example, the growing use of party drugs in the gay male community taxes existing mental health services (McDowell, 2000).[7] Many clients who utilize the services of CLCHC do not otherwise address these concerns with their medical doctor. The fact that substance abuse in the LGBT community was a recognized phenomenon did not mean that CLCHC was equipped to treat it. Substance abuse in the LGBT community is just one area that is ripe for research, and has been significantly under-examined in the psychiatric literature.[8] For a public health entity that relies on state and federal support for its solvency, the absence of a unified front in battling substance abuse and psychiatric pathology in the LGBT community has serious implications. The solidification of LGBT mental health as a field of study worthy of public health and research monies is necessary to understand fundamental LGBT health concerns, establish essential services, and attract and maintain mental health providers within the field.[9]

Today, Callen-Lorde continues to exemplify the spirit that led to the development of its predecessor, the Community Health Project. Though no longer an ad hoc team of health care providers volunteering in their off-hours to address the issues affecting the LGBT community, CLCHC now employs a staff of equally dedicated individuals to address the needs of that community. Their creativity and perseverance is helping to formulate the concept of LGBT health care for the future. Some of the CLCHC divisions described in this paper grew out of the inspiration of a few individuals. Developing and applying effective treatments for this diverse population make the field an intriguing one for medical and psychiatric disciplines. Clearly, the experience of the Callen-Lorde Community Health Center, and its predecessor, the Community Health Project, shows how bravely and diligently a community of healers can marshal around those that need scientific study, treatment and support.

NOTES

1. Similarly, during this time, mental health caregivers were not always accepting of the issues with which members of the LGBT population might present. Although the American Psychiatric Association had declassified homosexuality as a mental disorder in 1973, the repercussions of this decision had only begun to suggest that LGBT mental health care might be an area worthy of clinical study and research. Mental health care and crisis counseling for gays and lesbians were often provided by professionals who had been trained and supervised in environments that were often tolerant, at best, of LGBT-related issues.

2. It was named after Michael Callen, a gay man and founder of the People with AIDS (PWA) Coalition and of the Community Research Initiative, and Audre Lorde, the African-American educator and former New York State Poet Laureate who wrote extensively about her struggle with breast cancer.

3. Some key people involved in the growth of the program include Merle Cunningham, MD, a former Team leader and early founder of CHP, who continues as a member of the Board of Directors of the Callen-Lorde Health Center. Dr. Cunningham recalls the transition from a spirited, grass roots, volunteer-staffed "free clinic" to a fully licensed, state of the art medical practice that could meet New York State Health Department standards. He notes how a minimally supervised, but highly motivated staff molded itself into a financially solvent entity, while maintaining its unique accessibility to the community. Jeannetta Bushey, a clinical social worker, and the Director of Mental Health and Social Services, helped structure the mental health services at CHP, and then reconfigured them for the CLCHC facility. She recalls how everyone at CHP pulled together and contributed in some way, particularly in mental health emergencies. The severe space shortage at CHP fostered relationships amongst all the providers present that might not have otherwise formed. This would not be as readily preserved in the new facility, with different floors separating many of the clinical services previously provided in a single contiguous space. Privacy, rarely available at CHP, came at the cost of physical barriers that did not allow staff to see their peers very often in the new and spacious setting.

4. Steven Lee, MD, was the first psychiatrist to work at CLCHC through this program, followed by Khakasa Wapenyi, MD, in 2002. Both psychiatrists continued their work at CLCHC on a part-time basis at the conclusion of their fellowship years as part of the regular employed staff.

5. Though CLCHC ostensibly also operates on a sliding scale format for clients unable to pay the full amount, the scale is a "soft" one, and never results in anyone being turned away.

6. According to Marie Declet, the present Outreach Coordinator for the HOTT program.

7. Steven Lee noted that while 10% of gay men he evaluated had a substance abuse issue when he first worked at Callen-Lorde in 2000, that number jumped to a third or more three years later.

8. Editor's Note: See Guss, J.R. & Drescher, J., eds. (2000), *Addictions in the Gay and Lesbian Community*. New York: The Haworth Press.

9. Jeannetta Bushey recalls her own experience while working in the LGBT health care system: "Since there was little external validation for my work, I had to look more within and establish my own sense of value. This has certainly informed my current sense of competency."

REFERENCES

American Psychiatric Association (1974), Position statement on homosexuality and civil rights. *American J. Psychiatry*, 131:497.
American Psychiatric Association (1991), Position statement on HIV and youth. *American J. Psychiatry*, 148:1288.
American Psychiatric Association (1998), *Position statement on HIV and adolescents.* American Psychiatric Association Website *(http://www.psych.org/archives/980017. pdf)*.
American Psychiatric Association (2000), *Fact sheet: Gay, lesbian, bisexual issues.* American Psychiatric Association Website (http://www.psych.org/public_info/ gaylesbianbisexualissues22701.pdf).
Cabaj, R.P. & Stein, T.S., eds. (1996), *Textbook of Homosexuality and Mental Health.* Washington, DC: American Psychiatric Press.
The Harry Benjamin International Gender Dysphoria Association, Inc. (HBIGDA) (2001). HBIGDA website *(http://www.hbigda.org/)*.
LaBate, D.J. (1999), Unpublished letter to Jacqueline Elias, August 20. Michael Callen-Audre Lorde Health Center.
LaBate, D.J. (2000), Unpublished letter to Neal L. Cohen, May 17.
Michael Callen-Audre Lorde Health Center. Callen-Lorde website *(http://www.callen-lorde. org)*.
McDowell, D. (2000), Gay men, lesbians and substances of abuse and the "club and circuit party scene": What clinicians should know. *J. Gay & Lesbian Psychotherapy*, 3(3/4):37-57. Reprinted in: *Addictions in the Gay and Lesbian Community*, eds. J.R. Guss & J. Drescher. New York: The Haworth Press, 2002, pp. 37-57.
New Home for Gay/Lesbian Health Center (1997), *New York Times*, January 12.
Shilts, R. (1987), *And The Band Played On.* New York: St. Martin's Press.
Thompson, G. (1999), New clinics let lesbian patients be themselves; an effort to help a group that often shuns doctors. *The New York Times*, March 30.

Group Psychotherapy
for HIV-Positive Veterans
in a Veterans Administration Clinic

Michael Rankin, MD, MPH

SUMMARY. This paper describes the history of a psychotherapy group for HIV-positive veterans and service members on active military duty at a Veterans Administration clinic in Oakland, California, during the first decade of the epidemic. The author discusses the difficulties encountered working within a homophobic and AIDS phobic system, and the strategies used to make that work possible. *[Article copies available for a fee from The Haworth Document Delivery Service: 1-800-HAWORTH. E-mail address: <docdelivery@haworthpress.com> Website: <http://www. HaworthPress.com> © 2004 by The Haworth Press, Inc. All rights reserved.]*

KEYWORDS. AIDS, AIDS phobia, Department of Veterans Affairs, federal government, group psychotherapy, HIV, homophobia, public psychiatry, veterans

PROLOGUE

"How can it be" Fran demanded, "that here in the eye of the storm, in 1986, the fourth year of the AIDS epidemic, when my infectious disease clinic is

Michael Rankin is Clinical Professor of Psychiatry and Behavioral Sciences, George Washington University Medical School, Washington, DC (E-mail: NAVYDOCDC@ aol.com).

[Haworth co-indexing entry note]: "Group Psychotherapy for HIV-Positive Veterans in a Veterans Administration Clinic." Rankin, Michael. Co-published simultaneously in *Journal of Gay & Lesbian Psychotherapy* (The Haworth Medical Press, an imprint of The Haworth Press, Inc.) Vol. 8, No. 3/4, 2004, pp. 107-113; and: *Handbook of LGBT Issues in Community Mental Health* (ed: Ronald E. Hellman, and Jack Drescher) The Haworth Medical Press, an imprint of The Haworth Press, Inc., 2004, pp. 107-113. Single or multiple copies of this article are available for a fee from The Haworth Document Delivery Service [1-800-HAWORTH, 9:00 a.m. - 5:00 p.m. (EST). E-mail address: docdelivery@haworthpress.com].

Digital Object Identifer: 10.1300/J236v08n03_08

filled to overflowing with AIDS patients–how can it be that the Mental Health Clinic (MHC) is doing absolutely nothing for them?" It was my first day as chief of the Oakland, California, VA MHC; this feisty nurse, who would become a great ally, wanted me to fix the problem yesterday.

She needn't have been surprised that psychiatry and psychology were "doing absolutely nothing for them" in Oakland. We were doing little for HIV-positive veterans in any VA outpatient clinic in those days.

There were exceptions, of course in cities such as San Francisco, Los Angeles, and New York. Where gay, lesbian, and heterosexual clinicians demanded programs for these veterans, and where department and hospital chiefs supported them, the programs existed. Otherwise, veterans seeking care were urged to look elsewhere, even if they had no insurance and were eligible for VA care.

AIDS phobia was not limited to the Department of Veteran Affairs, of course. Members of President Clinton's Advisory Council on HIV and AIDS, arriving for a Council meeting in Washington, were checked through security by secret service agents wearing gloves.

STARTING THE GROUP

This paper presents a brief history of one HIV-support group in a clinic in Northern California during the first years of the epidemic. The paper will describe difficulties encountered by staff attempting to care for these veterans in a homophobic and AIDS phobic environment. It is a story that could be told about many if not most VA clinics in those days, and in some places even now.

The Oakland group began in 1986, as soon as I could get unpacked and learn my way around the clinic. I reviewed cases and potential referrals with Fran and the two internists who had chosen to work with this population; both were warm and empathetic physicians whose patients saw them as trusted advocates as well as knowledgeable clinicians.

We agreed that HIV-positive status would be the sole criterion for referral to the group. It would be open to gay, lesbian, and heterosexual veterans. Psychiatric diagnosis would be secondary, as long as the individual was capable of functioning in a group setting.

The nurse and physicians posted notice of the group in their offices and the waiting room; they encouraged everyone on their caseloads to attend. I could be trusted, they assured the skeptical veterans.

Eight men attended the first meeting, held from 2:30 to 4:00 p.m. in the MHC group room, a rather stark space badly in need of decoration. They and I negotiated the ground rules. It would be open to all HIV-positive veterans, not just to gay veterans, and not just to males. The group would meet once a week at 2:30, for an hour and a half. Nothing said in the group would leave the room. To the greatest extent possible, my chart notes would protect their privacy. Spouses and partners would be welcome only if they too were HIV-positive veterans.

Group members would have a say in the choice of a co-leader, if we ever had one. They also had the right to accept or reject trainees who might want to participate. I would provide chips, soft drinks, and juice at all sessions, and would "spruce up" the room.

We would begin each session with a brief "check in." Members could share as much biographical data as they liked, which gave them the opportunity at the first meeting to confirm what they had already heard–that I was gay, and though HIV negative, had already lost close friends and a former partner to AIDS.

Several of the rules would quickly change, beginning with the meeting time. The first gathering seemed to go well, but only two veterans came for the second. Those present weren't sure why the others were not there, so I called them. Two had decided it "just wasn't for them." Four felt uncomfortable in a waiting room with other veterans, certain everyone knew why they were there and looked down on them. They agreed to return if we changed the time to 5:00 to 7:30 p.m., when the waiting room would otherwise be empty.

The strategy worked. At the third meeting, we had six of the first selectees and two additions, one the partner of a member. It quickly became apparent that this was not a good thing for the group–the partners brought a dynamic that was not helpful, that was in fact destructive to the process. The man who insisted on being included if his partner was to participate did indeed have mild symptoms of depression. However, it quickly became clear that his primary concern was that his spouse might leave him for a man he met in the group.

I urged them to seek couples counseling with another staff member, which they agreed to do. One continued with the group, the other did not. We never again had two partners as members.

Despite an active outreach effort on my part and Fran's, no women veterans and no heterosexual veterans joined the group. It became all gay and all male by default. We began separate groups in the clinic for women, both heterosexual and lesbian, and for heterosexual veterans living with the virus, staffed by other clinicians. Neither was primarily HIV focused.

Diagnostically, most of the group met the criteria for adjustment disorders, though we also had members with mood disorders, alcohol and substance abuse, and early dementia. Several were combat veterans with mild post-traumatic stress disorder (PTSD). One had schizophrenia. It was touching to see how the group rallied around him, even when he was quite psychotic. They were much less patient with the few who were actively abusing drugs such as amphetamines and cocaine. These individuals were confronted and quickly left the group, referred to the clinic's substance abuse program.

THE SUPERVISOR

As word spread, more veterans demanded a place in the group. I started a waiting list, and considered beginning a second group. My senior supervisor, who arrived after I was hired by his predecessor, would have none of it. He flatly denied permission for an expansion of the program, insisting that I limit attendance to a few sessions at most, which I resisted, feeling a rigid time limit would destroy the group's effectiveness.

Nor was he eager to allow flexibility in my work schedule. Most clinic staff worked from 8 to 5; I was in the clinic until 8:00 p.m. on Tuesday evenings. VA policy allowed him to grant the flexibility; he did so with great reluctance. "Why are you wasting your time on 'those people,' " he demanded? "They're all going to die anyway."

He could not fire me for treating HIV-positive veterans, but he did have the authority to transfer me to a rural clinic in Redding, 200 miles north of Oakland; he had used the transfer strategy before with a psychiatrist who disagreed with him. At our supervisory meetings, he rarely failed to ask whether I would not prefer to live in a more "family oriented" community.

In retrospect, I believe my membership on the Board of Trustees of the San Francisco AIDS Foundation, and the fact that I chaired the National Committee on HIV and AIDS of Reform Judaism, and was thus, in his mind, "politically connected," kept him from moving me to Redding, or from discontinuing the group.

It probably didn't hurt that I was the only Vietnam combat veteran in his department, and that my primary work in the clinic was with Vietnam and other veterans with severe PTSD. A letter from an irate veteran to a member of Congress, complaining that his therapist had been snatched away, would not have enhanced the boss's career.

I found no reassurance in any of this. Nor could I appeal to my boss's supervisor, who was even more homophobic. It was difficult working with the threat of having to uproot my life in the San Francisco Bay area and move to a place where I knew no one.

Fortunately, after the 1992 election, and my appointment to the Presidents Advisory Council on HIV and AIDS, the issue became moot. From that time on, all mention of life in the country ceased.

Instead, the supervisor began hinting at favors I might obtain for him through my "contact" with the Clintons. Could I get him an autographed photograph of the President? I did, although I believe it was machine signed.

Would President Clinton like to jog with him the next time he was in the Bay Area? Perhaps the President would be interested in his thoughts about various issues, shared on a ride on Air Force One.

Remaining non-committal on those requests, I moved as quickly as I could during our supervisory sessions to issues of concern to the clinic. He was eventually promoted to a VA position of greater responsibility in another state, where he subsequently retired.

From conversations with VA colleagues at other centers, I learned that this lack of support–bordering on homophobic–was not unique to Oakland. It was typical in many VA hospitals and clinics, though it did get better toward the end of the 1990s, due in large measure to an excellent AIDS Coordinator at the Department of Veterans Affairs Central Office in Washington.

DEATH AND DYING

Despite the supervisor's opposition, the group continued to meet, with new members added as others left for various reasons. A few who joined were gay Navy and Army reservists who feared they would be discharged if they sought care at the region's military hospitals.

Death and dying issues were paramount in the first years. By 1989, half of the group's original members had died of AIDS. Most had felt themselves alienated from their families and from their faith communities, yet they wanted a service of remembrance, if not a sectarian funeral; they asked me to lead the service, which I did.

During their final illnesses, we had long discussions about readings and music they wanted at the service, and what those meant to them. These were the only individual sessions I had with group members. Typically I referred those with more severe psychopathology to MHC colleagues for individual therapy, allowing them to remain in the group as well.

Feeling increasingly stressed after three years as a solo group therapist, I invited a colleague from another mental health discipline to join me as co-leader, providing the group agreed. They grilled him mercilessly, then voted unanimously to accept him. Only then did they tell me they had been worried about me, and were glad I would have a "buddy" to co-lead the group.

Still later, a post doctoral psychology student joined the group as a trainee therapist, after gaining the group's approval. She remained for the year of her training, contributed greatly to the process, and was replaced by a second trainee when she left. A third trainee was rejected by the group because she insisted on taking notes during the sessions.

In a 1993 conversation with a friend, I bemoaned the fact that so many of these men lived on limited incomes in the inner city, mainly on disability payments–though a few still worked. They rarely had an opportunity to get out of the city–they could not afford a vacation. My friend offered his cabin at Pine Mountain Lake in the Sierras, near Yosemite, for a weekend outing, and offered his van as well. Another friend volunteered his home in Guerneville, a resort on the Russian River north of San Francisco. This was the beginning of a series of outings that added much to the group's morale, and to mine.

Every three or four months, we would leave on Friday afternoons for the lake or the river. My generous friends remained in the city–only group members could attend. We prepared meals together, watched videos, played cards, or just chatted after dinner. During the day, we hiked, rafted on the river, and picnicked in these beautiful settings. Once we walked through Yosemite Valley from Half Dome to Mirror Lake, pushing one of the group members in a wheel chair.

A favorite Sierra stopping point was the Iron Door Saloon, a restaurant and dance establishment in Groveland. Located a mile or two from Pine Mountain Lake, it was a weekend hangout for loggers and forest rangers, where country bands provided dance music for the men and their women friends. Invariably the men of the group would watch for an hour or so, then get up and dance with each other. Nobody seemed to mind; it was an accepting kind of place, as was the barber shop in Groveland. I noticed most of the men waited until our outings to get haircuts there, and finally asked why. "She's family," someone explained. "She won't let us pay her." Deciding where they got haircuts was not in my job description.

Another tradition was our Sunday morning breakfasts at the Ahwahnee at Yosemite and Fifes in Guerneville. They did let us pay.

The effect of these outings was amazing. I know they enhanced the lives of these men. I believe they prolonged them as well. Unfortunately, my co-therapist could not participate. His supervisor would not allow him to attend an event which, he said, was "probably mostly an orgy." Still, hoping for a ride on Air Force One, my supervisor declared himself indifferent to the trips, as long as I did not ask for compensatory time or VA funds.

As promising new medications were developed, the focus of the group changed from "when will I die?" to "what will I do now that I might live and I've retired, applied for disability, and sold my insurance?" It was a wonderful reordering of priorities, but the group was no less important to these men because of that reordering.

EPILOGUE

In December, 1996, I retired from the Veterans Administration. Another clinician joined as co-therapist, and the group continued for a few months. However, neither therapist had the necessary support from "the top," and in less than a year, the group disbanded. Members who needed it were referred for individual psychotherapy, or to other groups where AIDS was not the primary focus.

Six years later, living now in Arlington, Virginia, I remain in e-mail contact with several of the members. One has moved to Texas, another to Florida. Both report the situation in their respective VA clinics is much like what they experienced in Oakland in the early 1980s–services offered reluctantly, if at all. I understand the situation in some cities is much better now.

This, then, is what it was like to be a psychiatrist attempting to care for HIV-positive veterans in a homophobic system during the first decade of the epidemic. It wasn't an easy ten years, but I learned a great deal about practicing psychiatry in the public sector.

A good clinician can offer quality care in such institutions, but one must, above all, be comfortable with rigid bureaucracies, and have strategies for coping with these systems. Patient negotiation sometimes works; sometimes it does not. An ability to see the director's point of view, and to acknowledge the restraints under which s/he operates, is essential. Most bosses are not as prejudiced and unfeeling as mine was.

Still, there were times when the VA dictum "don't ask permission, just do it and plead for forgiveness later" seemed the only option. In rare cases, when everything else failed and the veteran was clearly being harmed, I let my patient know that nothing gets a VA clinic director's attention like a letter of inquiry from a member of Congress. There is a risk in using these strategies, however–one has to be willing to be fired for doing so. Yet, allowing a patient to be harmed by an absurd bureaucratic policy violated every ethical standard of my profession.

More than in private practice, it is necessary in the public sector to be comfortable in one's professional identity, and to enjoy, not just tolerate, working as part of a multidisciplinary team–no matter who heads the team. I found that comfort challenged, not by my psychology, social work, and nursing colleagues, but by clinic chiefs who referred to us as "providers," not physicians or clinicians.

This particular form of bureaucrat-speak felt offensive and condescending, whether it came from a non-clinician administrator or one with a health sciences degree. I lived with it, but I loved it when I heard a veteran tell an officious appointment clerk thirty years his junior "I don't have a 'provider,' I have a doctor and I need to see him. Where is he?"

Those years at the VA were the most challenging of my career, and also the most rewarding. It was an honor and a privilege to know the men of the group, and to work with colleagues such as Fran, Cliff, Nancy, Paula, and Matt.

They were, are, and always will be my heroes.

Being Gay and Mentally Ill:
The Case Study
of a Gay Man with Schizophrenia
Treated at a Community
Mental Health Facility

Michael C. Singer, PhD

SUMMARY. Gays and lesbians with major mental illness often spend their lives within the public mental health system, in which the existence of gay-affirmative programs is a rarity. This potentially alienating situation is often exacerbated by gaps in the training of psychodynamic clinicians that leave important issues of sexuality unexplored in most programs' core curricula. The Lesbian, Gay, Bisexual and Transgender (LGBT) Affirmative Program at the Heights Hill Mental Health Center in Brooklyn, New York is an exception to this common state of affairs.

This case presentation describes the two-year treatment of a gay man at the Center diagnosed with schizophrenia. An important portion of the therapeutic work was disentangling the two issues of the patient's minority status: being gay and mentally ill. At the beginning of treatment, the two categories were undifferentiated for him, and the difficulties of being gay were entangled with the difficulties of schizophrenia. Over

Michael C. Singer, PhD, is Adjunct Lecturer at Hunter College, Department of Psychology, 695 Park Avenue, New York, NY 10021 (E-mail: mcsinger@hunter.cuny.edu).

[Haworth co-indexing entry note]: "Being Gay and Mentally Ill: The Case Study of a Gay Man with Schizophrenia Treated at a Community Mental Health Facility." Singer, Michael C. Co-published simultaneously in *Journal of Gay & Lesbian Psychotherapy* (The Haworth Medical Press, an imprint of The Haworth Press, Inc.) Vol. 8, No. 3/4, 2004, pp. 115-125; and: *Handbook of LGBT Issues in Community Mental Health* (ed: Ronald E. Hellman, and Jack Drescher) The Haworth Medical Press, an imprint of The Haworth Press, Inc., 2004, pp. 115-125. Single or multiple copies of this article are available for a fee from The Haworth Document Delivery Service [1-800-HAWORTH, 9:00 a.m. - 5:00 p.m. (EST). E-mail address: docdelivery@haworthpress.com].

Digital Object Identifer: 10.1300/J236v08n03_09

time, the work to expand and clarify what it meant to be gay helped free the patient to explore the relationship between his sexuality and other components of his core identity.

Ultimately, the patient's notions about himself expanded and deepened: being gay took its place as one of his core attributes, but was not his only link to the outside world. The clinical work helped the patient to acquire more of a sense of his complexity as a human being, and just as important, a sense that being complex was normal. *[Article copies available for a fee from The Haworth Document Delivery Service: 1-800-HAWORTH. E-mail address: <docdelivery@haworthpress.com> Website: <http://www. HaworthPress.com> © 2004 by The Haworth Press, Inc. All rights reserved.]*

KEYWORDS. Community mental health center, countertransference, gay, homosexuality, mental health services, psychoanalytic psychotherapy, psychosis, public psychiatry, schizophrenia

INTRODUCTION

In July 1999, I began what would ultimately be a two-year clinical psychology externship at the Heights Hill Mental Health Center, a community outpatient program of South Beach Psychiatric Center, a New York State public mental hospital. Having completed a second-year externship at The New York Psychoanalytic Institute (NYPsI), I wanted to work with chronically ill patients, an experience that neither NYPsI nor my psychoanalytic doctoral program at suburban Adelphi University offered.

The Heights Hill Mental Health Center has an additional facility that particularly interested me: within the two floors of the clinic in downtown Brooklyn is a program intended specifically for severely mentally ill lesbian, gay, bisexual, and transgendered (LGBT) patients. This LGBT program is an integrated part of the larger clinic, but offers its patients the additional possibilities of working with gay and lesbian therapists and participating in various LGBT groups and social activities.

These gay-positive opportunities are not unusual in clinics that treat higher functioning, more affluent LGBT patients. However, they are virtually nonexistent for severely mentally ill patients, most of them poor and people of color, who have been in the public health system for a significant portion of their lives. The notion that a publicly operated mental health facility would regard these patients' sexuality as an important and affirmative part of their social and cultural identity was neither part of their prior experience, nor a situation that they had ever expected to encounter (Hellman, 1996).

Affirmative treatment for LGBT patients with major mental illness is often further compromised, because psychodynamic clinical psychology programs–

which train a significant proportion of the psychologists who work in New York–usually avoid open discussion of sexual diversity within their core curricula. As a result, psychologists frequently begin their professional careers with little understanding of the complex issues around variations of sexual identity, including their own emotional reactions to it (Singer, 2002). Working at Heights Hill was my own effort to gain some understanding of these issues.

The purpose of the following case presentation is to demonstrate some of the particular vulnerabilities of LGBT patients with major mental illness, and to examine some of the ways in which treatment can address the interaction between sexual minority status and major mental illness; in brief, to explain something of what I learned from two years at the Heights Hill Mental Health Center.

IDENTIFYING DATA

F was a foreign-born gay man in his 40s who had been at the clinic for two years prior to the beginning of this psychotherapeutic treatment. Diagnosed with undifferentiated schizophrenia and with additional obsessive/compulsive symptoms, F was monitored on a monthly basis by the LGBT program psychiatrist. Since coming to Heights Hill, he had been prescribed fluvoxamine (Luvox), 100 mg and olanzapine (Zyprexa), 7.5 mg hs. These dosages helped control the severity of F's symptoms. He was medication-compliant, but declined higher dosages because of side effects. He had been only inconsistently involved in therapy during this initial two-year period.

F had two presenting complaints: (a) he feared that men who spat on the streets and subway platforms were reacting to something bad about him, either that he was foreign or gay; and (b) he had a thought broadcasting delusion that caused him to feel very vulnerable in public places. F's two major obsessive compulsive symptoms included: (a) endlessly reordering the letters of written words, which made it difficult for him to understand what he read in books and magazines; and (b) standing for hours next to public trash cans reading the labels on discarded soda bottles, or as he put it, "reading garbage." When F read magazines on the subway, he heard a woman's voice emerge from the hum of the subway engine and berate him, in his native language, as a "stupid boy," usually for making mistakes in pronunciation or comprehension. While medication partially attenuated these symptoms, F's ability to develop relationships and his overall functioning were severely constrained.

THE FIRST YEAR

The initial work focused on the spitting, about which F seemed anxious to tell me. This seemed to be a good idea for several reasons: first, his fear of being spat at seemed to be related to his reluctance to leave his apartment for weekly sessions, and it was important to address this issue at the beginning of treatment; second, spitting seemed to have a private meaning for him that I wanted to understand as the first step of exploring what appeared to be his very personal and unusual use of language and symbolism.

Soon after treatment began, F and I began a detailed inquiry about spitting: we analyzed individual spitting events, we described the sounds of the spitting and its color, the trajectory and endpoint of the spit, and the demeanor and facial expression of spitters, as well as F's own actions at these times. F understood spitting as a reprimand or rejection, that "they were spitting on my heart." Later, he added that he had "cruised" some of these men, or simply made eye contact, having felt physically attracted to them and curious about how they felt toward him. Their spitting was a clear rebuke to his wanting to be close. F seemed angry and frustrated when he described these rejections. We searched together for meanings that made sense to both of us, a key activity when working psychotherapeutically with patients diagnosed with schizophrenia (Drescher, 1998).

Apparently understanding very little about his condition, F frequently asked about discontinuing his medication, since he noticed that his symptoms were improving. He attributed his mental illness to his immigration to the United States. When I told him that the medication and the therapy were helping to ease his symptoms, he was skeptical, and said he hoped to be normal someday and lead a normal life. His notion of normality seemed to hold meanings of which I was unaware.

The Entanglement of Sexual Diversity and Mental Illness

I wanted to understand how F conflated the two issues of his minority status: being gay and mentally ill. He claimed that he was comfortable with gayness; and in fact, he had sought out the LGBT program, and specifically requested a gay therapist. Both of these acts were considerable undertakings for someone with his limited interpersonal skills. F's being gay had been established, distinct, and identifiable for him since before his immigration to the US, and his wide reading of the gay popular press had helped him feel some genuine acceptance of his sexuality. He went to gay pride parades in several boroughs of New York City each year. Yet, his spitting delusion suggested that he had some pejorative associations to–and uncomfortable feelings about–being gay. His family had always been angrily critical of his sexuality; and his few sexual relationships of any duration had been deeply unsatisfying, even humiliating experiences.

On the other hand, F had no notion of the meaning of being diagnosed with schizophrenia, especially in the concrete sense of how it had affected his ability to lead a satisfying life. He attributed the near hopelessness of finding a partner, or even a close gay friend, to the vicissitudes of gay life, rather than to the isolating effects of his mental illness. The two categories were undifferentiated for him, and the difficulties of being gay were mixed up with the difficulties of schizophrenia. What the two categories had in common was that both placed him in a minority position and increased his sense of vulnerability. F's non-understanding was perhaps part of what was expressed by his spitting fantasy: He was punished by isolation for being different from other people in some essential, yet unknowable way.

Initial Countertransference Issues

At the beginning of the treatment, my confusion during our sessions mirrored F's own. I felt overwhelmed by his needs and suffocated by his desire for closeness. F stood too close to me at the beginning of sessions; he moved his chair uncomfortably nearer to mine as each session progressed; and he seemed to be so immediately dependent on my reactions during sessions that his speech became almost incomprehensible whenever I turned a page of my note pad.

I imagined that F's approach was a sexual one, the attraction of a gay man to another man, but this was my own naive attempt to normalize my experience with him so that I could understand it better. At the time, I failed to appreciate his more primitive fears of merger. With his paranoid symptomatology and no close relationships of any kind, F had no way to understand a supportive or safe relationship with a therapist or any other person, and was, it seemed, experiencing our first meetings as a loss of boundaries.

To ease my own considerable anxiety about our boundaries, my supervisor suggested that I could occasionally comment on the uniqueness of the therapeutic relationship and its particular quality of closeness in a once-a-week setting. This mantra granted me an illusion of control and calmness at a time when I was experiencing very little of either.

As we worked out these initial issues, F developed his own repetitive statement that seemed to help him manage his anxiety. He began many of his explanations and stories by asking me, "You're gay, right?" When I asked him about this, he responded that my being gay made it easier for me to understand the things that happened between men and that neither of us would be embarrassed. He always laughed after this explanation.

Beyond F's obscure clarification, his repeated use of the question seemed to have additional meaning. First, he used it as an incantation, a reminder to himself that it was safe to proceed on this intimate journey with me. He told me that he had never spoken to anyone else about the things that we were exploring. By asking the question, "Are you really gay?" he seemed to be playing with his own notions of object permanence, wondering, "Are you still the same? Are you still there for me?" This rephrasing of the question, to which he returned later in the treatment, also referred back to his own accomplishment in having found this gay-friendly clinic and having had the courage to ask for a gay therapist. Part of his disbelief at the beginning of treatment had been that, after 25 years in the public health system, a general psychiatric clinic would have honored his gayness enough to have a category of therapists who were actually gay and whom one could request. These are some of the meanings we began to create.

Over the months, this expansion and clarification of what it meant to be gay helped F feel free to play with it in our sessions. Winnicott (1971) remarked that playing has a place and a time, although it is neither internal nor a part of the purely external world. He explained, "To control what is outside one has to do things, not simply to think or to wish, and doing things takes time. Playing is doing."

Our play around this growing and differentiating notion of being gay was perhaps a special case of play. We began with an attribute from F's inner reality and acted on it so that it became imbued with the quality of something in the world, an anchor, a given, something normal and tangible that he could share with me when so many other things were unpleasant or unstable. As individuals, being gay represented something different for each of us, with our different personal and even idiosyncratic symbolizations. In the treatment, however, we were creating a shared narrative that described what it meant to be gay, while also teasing apart and examining F's experience of rejection and punishment. Drescher (1998) suggests that this collaborative search for co-created meanings, which is a natural byproduct of psychoanalytic psychotherapy, can transform work with patients diagnosed with schizophrenia into hopeful enterprises. In fact, F experienced this core portion of our work together as helpful and enormously constructive.

F's involvement in the treatment deepened and he began to reflect on the work we were doing together. Near the end of the first year he said, "You know, Michael, this study of the spitting we've done has been very important." We were then able to move on.

THE SECOND YEAR

While it is beyond the scope of this article to examine the particular vulnerability of persons with major mental illness to HIV infection, this connection has been extensively documented in recent years (e.g., McKinnon, Cournos and Herman, 2002; Stoskopf, Kim and Glover, 2001). F had never been tested for HIV, although he had engaged in unprotected sex with several partners, most of whom were anonymous, and at least one of whom had died from AIDS. One of my goals had been for F to be tested for HIV. Near the end of the first year of treatment, F tested positive for HIV and learned that he had AIDS.

In the weeks after hearing the news, F was anxious and destabilized. While our previous work and strong connection mitigated this distress, he was once again troubled by his symptoms, which seemed to portend renewed isolation. His speech was disorganized, and his skin red and blotchy.

The treatment team at the clinic was worried about F's ability to go through this crisis without decompensating. In particular, I feared that if I did not find some way to help him focus on the reality of his health crisis, both its challenges and opportunities, then the notion of being contaminated and worthless could overwhelm his limited ability to handle bad feelings through disavowal and projection. Nevertheless, F had begun to talk about his "death sentence" and his "useless life," and this indicated to me that he was making a concerted effort to come to terms with his profound grief and anger.

For my own part, I felt inadequate and frightened about failing F at such a difficult time, and also responsible for having suggested the HIV testing in the first place. Once again, as at the beginning of the treatment, my own difficult feelings paralleled his own, and I tried to use them in a constructive way.

I altered the frame of our sessions so that at least part of each was devoted to speaking about F's reactions. We explored his intense grief, mourning, and anxiety; and also dealt with equally complicated practical matters, such as medication, prognosis, and finding a good medical clinic and support group that could respond to the special needs of a gay patient with schizophrenia and AIDS. This steady exploration and problem-solving of concrete issues helped F get through a very difficult period and take control of his treatment. Its aftermath included a significant change in his life: an enormous increase in the number of people with whom F needed to interact regularly. Infectious disease physicians, nurse practitioners, AIDS support groups, and a whole array of ancillary personnel took their places in his world. We spent a great deal of time figuring out how F could navigate this new, highly social life style.

Over the next months, F established a new equilibrium and began to settle back into the treatment. That the therapy survived and F remained relatively stable encouraged a further deepening of our relationship. He began to talk about other times in his life when he had felt hopeless, especially during his first breakdown during adolescence.

Exploring the Physicalized Interior

F explained that he had suffered from thoughts that got stuck inside his head and then were lost, especially thoughts about anger and humiliation that were the most difficult for him to put into words. He meant this in a physical sense. He said his breakdown occurred because so many bad thoughts had gotten stuck and lost that they took up all the space inside his body. He couldn't move or communicate. He had felt as if bloated by poison, with swollen joints and a swollen brain. F lay paralyzed on the floor of his room for two days until his brother took him to the hospital. F said these losses still occurred and were very upsetting. I suggested that together we watch for thoughts that got stuck or lost during his sessions to see what we could understand about them.

I did not imagine that we could really get to the root of these losses of focus, since they were probably the result of an unknowable combination of his mental illness, neurological impairment, and medication side effects. But we had been given an opportunity to observe and explore more deeply how he experienced his own emotional life and the factors that impinged on it.

F began to let me know when he lost a thought. At first this happened only occasionally, every few sessions, at which times he would anxiously blurt out, "Michael, I lost my idea!" We would retrace our steps, trying to find where he had gotten lost, and then how.

Although a typical pattern never emerged in the nature of his "lost thoughts," we did discover something of the circumstances in which they became lost. The system F created to carry on this investigation was highly physicalized: thoughts, feelings, and ideas seemed to acquire physical substance. Whether or not F was able to retrieve or reconstruct a lost train of thought, he could always describe the feeling as it bounced around, ricocheting against various parts of his head, jamming into fissures, crowding out other thoughts, hidden in shadow, and ultimately either retrieved or not.

If a thought was irretrievable, he would move on, disappointed. However, when his search was successful, F was very happy and we engaged in a brief celebratory cheer before he continued on his way. We had created an energized, personalized, metaphorical language: the description of physical sensations caused by different kinds of flying thoughts.

In retrospect, this strange pinball game was closely related to F's thought broadcasting worries: when thoughts take on physical existence, as his had done, it is not so difficult to imagine that other people can see them. Having accepted this notion, the possibility of hurling angry thoughts at another person in the form of spit barely seems to represent a further stretch of one's imagination, except in the attribution of pain-causing abilities to spitting.

Anger and Idealization

Our prior work had established sufficient trust for F to explore how he became anxious and how he dissociated his unpleasant feelings. He approached this part of the treatment with a kind of loosening up of his inhibitions regarding anger. He told me about times that he had spit at other people in anger. He described how he fought with his relatives. He railed against his doctors. He was making progress.

During this time, F began traveling around New York City searching for AIDS doctors and support groups. He now rode the subway without restraint. F had become dissatisfied with his nurse practitioner at the medical clinic, whom he angrily accused of withholding information. He joined several AIDS support groups, and some of their members advised him to find a more responsive medical clinic. F seemed unable to pick and choose from the advice given him, trying instead to follow all of it uncritically. He was experiencing many changes in his life and this made him feel frustrated and angry.

While F had never directly expressed anger toward me, I suspected that I was evoking similar feelings, but that his idealization of me made it difficult for him to be open about his anger. Yet, his loss of one or two thoughts in every session and his increasing success connecting with other difficult feelings seemed to be paving the way.

When I asked him about this anger, he said that it was inappropriate to be angry with me because we were so close and he did not want to ruin the relationship. I told him that even people who were very close like us could get angry and at each other and that understanding this anger could deepen our relationship.

At the beginning of the treatment, this concept would have been inconceivable to a man who had experienced lifelong neglect and abuse. Even at this point, F responded skeptically; yet, he seemed able to talk about the possibility that anger might be better dealt with by expression than by being trapped inside his head. He was certainly able to recognize anger and anxiety when he experienced them, without an immediate dissociation.

During this period, I had felt increasingly pressured by F to be focused during our sessions, as if he had so many things to think about that keeping track of his thoughts was unimportant. My experience was that F's disordered thoughts, what I might have referred to as his psychotic process, was growing stronger and beginning to dominate whatever "keeping track" I imagined I was doing for both of us. In my own malaise, drowning in ideas, I experienced a powerlessness that resembled F's description of his first breakdown. He was communicating his anger to me, without the need for words, or spitting. In contrast, I was aware of my increasing passivity, and I was less able to connect as our sessions went on. It seemed that F had succeeded in making his thought broadcasting a reality, allowing me to directly share his experience of helplessness, while removing meaning from our spoken words.

One day, the inevitable happened and I lost one of my own thoughts. It did not bounce around, as F's did. Rather, it seemed to burst gently, like a bubble, and disappear. The sensation was not unpleasant. "F, I've lost a thought," I said.

F became enraged, berating me, expressing his general disgust with my incompetent provocation, and mimicking me sardonically when I tried to speak. It was not until several weeks had elapsed that he could begin to talk about his towering anger. I had failed him by having limitations that left him staring at his own thought disorder after he had tried so hard to erase it. My failure had held up a mirror; yet, I had contained his anxiety enough for him to experience this anger toward me without dissociation. We had been through a moment of powerful trial and empathy.

F and I were very much alike at that moment: human, gay, and imperfect. An enormous weight of almost two years' duration had been lifted from my shoulders and I felt relieved.

A FINAL QUESTION, AND TERMINATION

Our second year, filled with challenge and discovery, drew to a close. F spoke more freely about anger in his sessions, and how he had expressed it toward me. However, he could not admit that this had had any salutary effect. We explored his grief over our impending termination, and what the end of the treatment meant to each of us. F began many of his comments during termination with the question, "I'm normal, right, like you?" When I asked him about this, he replied, "You know, normal, except that I take medication." After all we had been through, this was a trickier question to answer than it would have been two years earlier.

His notions about himself had expanded and deepened over the years: being gay had taken its place as one of his core attributes, but was no longer the only circumstance we shared, or his only safe link to the outside world.

F's feelings about being gay were still highly ambivalent, but now there were many separate factors that comprised this ambivalence: the social stigma that he experienced as a gay man in his immigrant community; his lack of friends with whom he could be "out;" the psychological stress of AIDS; and finally, the chronic mental illness that heightened his experience of difference and isolation. We had begun to name and explore each of these aspects during treatment. And while he would likely examine the interaction between being gay and mentally ill for the rest of his life, for the most part he no longer attributed his extreme social isolation or his thought disorder to his sexuality.

F had looked deeply at his delusions and, at the end of the treatment, had even seen his thought disorder mirrored in me. We had explored many parts of his life, and he had ultimately been able to achieve a connected relationship. Our work had helped him to acquire more of a sense of his complexity as a human being, and just as important, a sense that being complex was normal. He had also discovered hope.

F's mental illness will most likely always be with him. It will always interact in a complicated way with the rest of his personality, including his being gay, his intelligence and curiosity, his generosity of spirit, and his HIV status. He also seemed to acknowledge that his more "normal" parts would help him deal with the challenges from the parts "that needed medication."

REFERENCES

Drescher, J. (1998), Discussion of Andrew Lotterman's "Psychotherapeutic techniques with schizophrenic patients." William Alanson White Society Scientific Colloquium, New York, NY, October 21.

Hellman, R.E. (1996), Issues in the treatment of lesbians and gay men with chronic mental illness. *Psychiatric Services*, 47:1093-1098.

McKinnon, K., Cournos, F. & Herman, R. (2002), HIV among people with chronic mental illness. *Psychiatric Quarterly*, 73:17-31.

Singer, M.C. (2002), Reenfranchising psychoanalysis. *Psychoanalytic Psychology*, 19:167-181.

Stoskopf, C.H., Kim, Y.K. & Glover, S.H. (2001), Dual diagnosis: HIV and mental illness, a population-based study. *Community Mental Health Journal*, 37: 469-479.

Winnicott, D.W. (1971), *Playing and Reality*. New York: Routledge.

Treatment
of a Transgender Client with Schizophrenia
in a Public Psychiatric Milieu:
A Case Study by a Student Therapist

Noel R. Garrett, MA

SUMMARY. This case presentation discusses an unusual clinical experience for a psychology student in training. It addresses the role of gender identity in the treatment of a transgender person with major mental illness receiving care in a public psychiatric milieu.

The example here describes one of a few open male-to-female individuals on the caseload of the milieu. The client regularly discussed her view that she had not been understood in prior therapy settings, all of which have been public psychiatric facilities. Working with this patient provided a glimpse into an unusual system where the gender identity component was relevant to the overall planning and execution of treatment.

Lesbian, gay, bisexual, and transgender (LGBT) individuals may be resistant to disclose details of their sexual identity to therapists in public settings for fear of being rejected, abandoned, or further diagnosed as sexually deviant. While most public psychiatric facilities have diverse

Noel R. Garrett, MA, is Doctoral Candidate at the New School University, New York, NY.

Address correspondence to: Noel R. Garrett (E-mail: noelrgarrett@yahoo.com).

[Haworth co-indexing entry note]: "Treatment of a Transgender Client with Schizophrenia in a Public Psychiatric Milieu: A Case Study by a Student Therapist." Garrett, Noel R. Co-published simultaneously in *Journal of Gay & Lesbian Psychotherapy* (The Haworth Medical Press, an imprint of The Haworth Press, Inc.) Vol. 8, No. 3/4, 2004, pp. 127-141; and: *Handbook of LGBT Issues in Community Mental Health* (ed: Ronald E. Hellman, and Jack Drescher) The Haworth Medical Press, an imprint of The Haworth Press, Inc., 2004, pp. 127-141. Single or multiple copies of this article are available for a fee from The Haworth Document Delivery Service [1-800-HAWORTH, 9:00 a.m. - 5:00 p.m. (EST). E-mail address: docdelivery@haworthpress.com].

Digital Object Identifer: 10.1300/J236v08n03_10

caseloads, it appears that LGBT issues, specifically those of transgender individuals, may not be receiving the level of attention required to provide appropriate treatment to this population. *[Article copies available for a fee from The Haworth Document Delivery Service: 1-800-HAWORTH. E-mail address: <docdelivery@haworthpress.com> Website: <http://www.HaworthPress. com> © 2004 by The Haworth Press, Inc. All rights reserved.]*

KEYWORDS. Community mental health center, cross-dressing, gender identity disorder, GID, homosexuality, LGBT, mental health, mental health services, psychiatry, psychosis, psychotherapy, public psychiatry, public sector, schizophrenia, transgender, transsexual

IDENTIFYING DATA

This is the case of M, a 48-year-old, single, African-American, male-to-female (MTF) preoperative transsexual. M was referred to an urban, public, outpatient psychiatric treatment facility by a local gay community services center after being discharged from a state mental health facility following a recent psychiatric hospitalization. M identified as being transgender, and used the feminine gender in addressing her personal concerns and issues. She resided alone in an apartment sponsored by a Christian counseling organization, was supported on social security benefits and had Medicaid coverage for her health care.

M stands nearly six feet two inches tall, and weighs approximately 190 to 200 pounds. M attended most early sessions neatly dressed and groomed in female attire consisting of a black dress, high-heeled shoes, and a shoulder-length wig, usually with a small knit hat. M generally wore makeup, and appeared preoccupied with her overall feminine appearance. In later sessions, M presented in male attire, but still carried a purse. On occasion, when male attired, M would wear minimal makeup, but remained preoccupied with her appearance.

PSYCHIATRIC HISTORY

M has a significant psychiatric history and entered the public sector following her first psychiatric decompensation. She had a history of multiple, extensive psychiatric hospitalizations since the age of eighteen. Initially, M was unable to report any relevant details regarding early admissions. However, during the course of treatment, M began to disclose that her first admission followed her discharge from the Marine Corps. While still in the Marines, she developed an overwhelming and obsessional need to write, stopping at any time to open her notebook and jot down all of her thoughts. During one inspection in the presence of her drill sergeant and fellow marines, this need intensified. She reached into her footlocker, removed her journal, and began to write her thoughts down. This went on for some time as her drill sergeant tried to get her attention. When she "came to," as she put it, the sergeant demanded that she read to the entire platoon what she had written. Embarrassed, she followed orders. She was subsequently discharged after two months of boot camp.

Shortly thereafter, M began to hear voices and became delusional. The voices convinced her that she had been destined to die like Christ to save the world, but could no longer fulfill this destiny after being caught for shoplifting at age 12. Instead of relieving the suffering of the world, she would have to suffer instead. She feared this and tried to kill herself. She was admitted to a hospital and diagnosed with schizophrenia. Despite the suicide attempt, she denied being depressed, and was treated with haloperidol (Haldol) and benztropine (Cogentin).

M was next hospitalized in her 30s after cutting her wrists in response to stressors focused on her transgender identity. Later hospitalizations were associated with psychotic features, including paranoid ideation. She differentiated the conviction that people were following her during these episodes from non-psychotic thoughts at other times about people critically judging her for being transgendered. M was unable to provide exact dates of past hospitalizations, but reported that her third hospitalization was in response to a second suicide attempt associated with auditory hallucinations. She was treated with thiothixene (Navane) and discharged to a local public mental health center for psychotherapy in December 1990, where she continued treatment from January 1991 to May 1995. M recalled motivation to stay in treatment at that time in order to prevent further relapses.

M's next hospitalization occurred in 2000 while she was in the process of completing course work toward an associate's degree in optometry at a local community college. Although she had received excellent grades, despite her many fears, M reported having difficulty in two required mathematics courses. She was not consistently taking her medication while attending school, and when this produced no immediate ill effects, she stopped taking the medication altogether. As pressure to complete her course work increased, she again began hearing voices and felt "out of control." M became disorganized, and fell behind on rent payments and other financial obligations. She was evicted from her apartment and subsequently picked up from the street by the police. She was involuntarily hospitalized for two months.

A subsequent hospitalization occurred in July, 2001, three months after being physically attacked by a group of men in her neighborhood. Information from hospital records and her residential program case manager indicated that

M had become increasingly confused and withdrawn, and had active suicidal ideation during the three-month period preceding the hospitalization. She became isolated, selectively mute, anhedonic, anorexic with weight loss, and was unable to manage her daily activities. She was hospitalized by the case manager, and was discharged in August, 2001 with a diagnosis of schizophrenia and depressive disorder, not otherwise specified (NOS). She was treated with sertraline (Zoloft) and thiothixene, but soon denied any depression and discontinued the antidepressant. Diphenhydramine (Benadryl) was prescribed for insomnia.

Following the attack, M no longer felt safe in her neighborhood as a transgender person. In fact, she was convinced that people, in general, did not accept her as the person she was. To address these concerns, M requested assignment to a transgender therapist. After nearly two months of effort, initial contact was made with the current community mental health center program, and treatment began in August, 2001.

M reported minor post-traumatic symptoms in response to the attack that precipitated the hospitalization. She questioned the need for medication, but agreed to adhere to her regimen of thiothixene, 5 mg and diphenhydramine 50 mg. M also received hormone therapy from a public health clinic, consisting of spironolactone 25 mg and estradiol 2 mg.

M had no history of alcohol abuse, but reported using small amounts of marijuana when engaging in sexual relations. She drank one beer a month, usually with dinner. She denied any psychiatric history in her family, or any history of physical or sexual abuse as a child.

M was diagnosed with the *DSM* diagnoses of (1) Schizophrenia, (2) a "rule/ out" of Major Depressive Disorder, Recurrent, with Psychotic Features, (3) Gender Identity Disorder, and (4) Adjustment Disorder (American Psychiatric Association, 1994). Although she was clearly traumatized by the recent physical attack, M did not meet formal diagnostic criteria for Post-Traumatic Stress Disorder.

PERSONAL HISTORY

M was born in the Southern US, a fraternal twin, who was the youngest of four children. M's twin sister died shortly after birth of unknown causes. M reported that her mother became cold and distant following the death of the child, but was still someone she could turn to when M was harassed by her oldest sister. M's father died when she was an infant. Her mother died when M was in the seventh grade. M moved to New York and was raised by her oldest sister when they could no longer afford the housing expenses. This is when she first recalled feeling "different," and when her social discomfort began. M talked of this time as a disturbing period. She missed her friends down South, with whom she imagined growing up and spending her life.

Even as a young child, M "loved putting on women's clothing." She would sneak into her sister's room and try on her clothes. In junior high school, M cross-dressed more frequently. She recalled an instance in her teens when her sister returned home while M was wearing her clothing. Upon hearing her sister enter the house, M quickly removed the clothes, but was humiliated when she had to walk through the house naked to reach her own room. Her sister subsequently placed a lock on her bedroom door and forbade M from wearing her clothes. M believed this experience instilled the conviction that "regular" people despise "irregular" transgender (and other LGBT) individuals. Her desire to cross dress remained strong, but M kept this aspect of her life hidden until much later in her life.

M reported frequent harassment for being effeminate while growing up. Attracted to men, she was initially confused and thought she was gay, but later began to see herself more as a woman attracted to men. At age 48, M reported that she "wanted to live as a transgender person full time," and decided to relinquish her masculine identity. Simultaneously, she reported this experience to be "difficult," and questioned the motives of others in their harassment and overall dislike of "people like [her]."

M graduated from high school, and later attended college with excellent grades. But she dropped out just prior to receiving her associate's degree because of difficulty passing algebra and trigonometry. She did not return to school, and lost interest in completing the degree. She began to pursue her desire to become a writer, composing poetry, copyrighting her work, and sending it to various contests and publishers. M has had no significant employment history, and is supported on SSI.

M had little contact with remaining family members, not wanting them to know how badly she was doing. Her oldest brother and sister resided in the Southwest. Another brother lived in the South. M remained in New York City living a lonely life "because people don't understand my transgenderism." She reported no close friendships, but expressed the desire to increase her transgender social network.

M frequently acknowledged that having a mental illness as a transgender person stood in her way. She referred to her "double-stigma" as something that separated her from everyone else. She was convinced that no one, not even other transgender people, could understand the hatred she experienced. She felt "most at home" in a feminine role, but hesitated to meet others, fearing rejection for being mentally ill.

COURSE OF TREATMENT

Initially, M was quiet and guarded. It was not clear whether she would continue with treatment when informed her therapist was not transgender; finding a transgender therapist had been her most important goal. She asked numerous questions related to transgender concerns, seeming to test her new therapist's awareness of, and sensitivity to the issues she raised. As the course of treatment progressed, she indicated that he had apparently "passed the test."

M rarely discussed symptoms of her mental illness, including her multiple hospitalizations. She felt that she had been misdiagnosed. But any attempt at exploration was met with dismissal, a defense that became prominent throughout the course of treatment. On a few occasions, however, she discussed her "double-stigma," providing the opportunity to explore these experiences, if only briefly.

M always presented as neatly dressed and groomed, usually wearing traditional woman's clothing. During initial sessions, M made very little eye contact. Her speech was soft and slow, and she carefully enunciated all of her words as if to impress the listener with her eloquence and stereotypic femininity. She believed others were continuously observing her, judging her poise and feminine behaviors.

She arrived for sessions holding a cosmetic sponge to blot her lip. On many occasions, usually several in a single session, M spoke of "this problem" of lip perspiration which began in childhood when playing with her girlfriends. M's lip would perspire, and they would comment, "Look, M is watering [his] mustache again." M never forgot this, and became convinced that, as a female, she must be more vigilant to prevent humiliation in front of others. She was dismayed that it drew unnecessary and unwelcome feedback. In response, she developed a strategy of blotting her lip so that other people would recognize that she was aware of it. She rationalized that her actions would make it less uncomfortable for "them."

Initial sessions were somewhat confusing, as M would discuss both her male and female identities in a manner that implied they were two separate and distinct entities. For example, when discussing the time she was assaulted, she would comment about going out as *Mark*, and compared it to going out as *Maria*. She indicated that *Mark* would never be approached or criticized by others, whereas *Maria* was forever fending off negative and harassing comments by others. M appeared either unaware or unphased that a person of her stature would have significant difficulty "passing" as a woman. She rejected any interpretation of her surprised response when others expressed their ignorance of those who were different. As *Mark*, she was more assertive; as *Maria*, she would prompt herself that "Women don't do that. Women don't fight." There appeared to be a complete split between these two seemingly discrete identities. But, with time, M began to accept that *Mark* and *Maria* were aspects of a single person.

M shared details about important events in her life at a very superficial level. For example, at the time of one hospitalization, she became homeless and lost all of her personal possessions. She reported this in a very matter-of-fact way, dismissing her feelings of loss with, "It doesn't matter." Similarly, she minimized her own feelings, both as *Mark* and *Maria*, when talking about the physical attack. Attempts to explore her transgender concerns and how they affected her life were met with this same defensive response.

M began to explore more of the interpersonal stresses in her immediate environment. After the physical attack, she began to understand how dubious she was as to whether becoming *Maria* was a good idea or not. She also realized how ambivalent she had been about relocating to a new apartment. She wanted to make friends in the community, but had no idea how to pursue this. She quickly dismissed the possibility of clubs and bars, stating, "Those people just do drag for entertainment–they're not transgender." A common theme was concern about having to go out as *Mark* while yearning to go out more often as *Maria*.

About three months into her treatment, a transgender support group was organized at the clinic and M was invited to participate. She was excited that other transgender people would be attending. M and her therapist discussed how this could be a good forum to discuss her concerns regarding socialization and acceptance. She had previously attended support groups at the local LGBT Community Center, but stopped because she could not always go as *Maria*, and feared that others would not accept her in her masculine identity. M reiterated her early conviction that being transgendered was "irregular," and, therefore, she could not be part of the world of "regular" people. However, she was able to consider that being transgendered was different for many people, and that in reality, she was still a person. This knowledge, however, had no obvious impact on her acceptance of her sexual identity.

After eight months in treatment, M started coming to sessions dressed in masculine attire, but did not disclose her reasons for doing so. She still carried a purse, patted her lip with a cosmetic sponge, and emphasized her explanation of why this occurs. It was clear that M's appearance–dressed in masculine attire, but carrying her purse–generated attention, but this attention was now directed at *Mark*, rather than *Maria*. M attended the support group in male attire as well. She raised questions regarding other participants' comfort level in identifying as transgender. This seemed to reassure her, and eventually, M returned to female attire. Soon after, she announced to the group that she had decided to transition into living her life as a female, "one hundred percent of the time." She appeared very confident about this decision, and presented on the outside, and to all appointments at the clinic as *Maria*. Her mood became more euthymic, and she appeared more assured about her plans and goals for the future.

After a few months, however, she suddenly began to present as *Mark* again, and stopped coming to the support group. This time, an explanation was forthcoming. M had been assigned to a new counselor at her residential program, a self-identified "Christian counselor" who encouraged her to return to Bible study. One day, M posed a question that changed the direction of therapy sessions: "Can a transsexual person who did everything according to God be saved?" When M first asked herself this question, she opened the Bible randomly. A passage highlighted in red stated, "Neither do I condemn thee you, go forth and sin no more." M took this as, "I forgive you for sinning, be *Mark*, and don't do it again." Subsequent sessions focused on determining if the Bible was being used to generate answers to her questions, or whether this passage may have triggered her fears of being "irregular." It became apparent that M had concretely interpreted the passage, neglecting the context in which it was presented. It was *Mark* who read the passage and not *Maria*, which further complicated its interpretation.

Shortly afterwards, a new residential counselor was assigned who was more open to M's transgender concerns. Almost immediately, she returned to her discussion of her conflicted transgenderism. She expressed remorse that, at the request of her previous counselor, she had donated all of her female clothing and accessories to a charity for homeless women. She acknowledged that her transgender desire was still very strong, and that she missed being *Maria*. She reported that she was unable to dress as *Maria* because she had no clothing.

M returned to the concern of having "a double stigma" because of her psychiatric diagnosis and transgender status. Because she had rarely discussed her psychiatric illness in previous sessions, this comment seemed almost incongruent with the trend of recent thoughts. M now denied psychosis, and focused on depressive symptoms, but rationalized these as the result of other people's behavior toward her. She believed her troubles from the past would be "erased" if she could just live her life as a transgender person. She believed her mental illness was secondary to the complexity and challenges of her transgender identity, and that her illness would "go away" if she could live her life as *Maria*. Efforts to question this assumption were dismissed.

M began to disclose early memories, and these brought into focus some of the issues that arose during the earlier course of treatment. One, for example, had to do with her selection of a female name. M was born a twin, and her sister's name was *Maria*. M believed she would be able to obtain her sister's birth certificate and live her life as *Maria* with "legal documentation." She was certain that she could change her identity to that of her deceased twin sister legally, and make a fresh start for herself, free of current debt, mental illness, and issues of being "irregular." By doing so, she thought she could leave her problems behind and start anew. With further exploration, M reluctantly admitted that she was still responsible for past circumstances in her life, and that changing her identity did not excuse her of responsibilities such as previous debt.

M continued to question her transgender identity. She had regularly expressed a desire to relocate through her residential program to a neighborhood that was more accepting of her lifestyle. She became increasingly isolated and withdrawn, and missed several sessions without contacting her therapist to cancel appointments. Attempts to contact her were left unanswered, but eventually M responded, explaining that she had taken herself to the hospital after becoming increasingly paranoid. On discharge, she returned to therapy. Hospital records noted symptoms on admission of delusional perceptions variously consisting of personal messages from the television, or, for example, seeing a bald person, which "meant" that she should cut her hair off. She also had auditory hallucinations–loud and clear voices outside her head when no one was around, telling her to leave the neighborhood. She acknowledged that she had not been taking her medication regularly.

DISCUSSION

M's initial requirement for a transgender therapist was anxiety-provoking to the author, a student therapist, because it raised issues of therapist self-disclosure. This became a focal point in supervision sessions. To encourage M to return to treatment, while providing a safe and understanding space in which to develop a good therapeutic alliance, the dictum that the therapist remain relatively anonymous seemed inappropriate. It would have been disconcerting and upsetting to M if her initial requirement had been ignored. It felt as though the patient had set the foundation for the frame of therapy, and her therapist experienced a sense of vulnerability and confusion. This was resolved by exploring therapist reactions to the accumulating interactions with M, and understanding her predictable patterns and limited capacity for objective, mindful reflection. McWilliams (1994) says, "Psychotic people are so desperate for basic human relatedness and for hope that someone can relieve their misery that they are apt to be deferential and grateful to any therapist who does more than classify and medicate them." Understanding M, and not merely classifying her as a psychotic patient, had significant positive implications in her treatment.

Initial sessions focused on transgender issues only, with little, if any, discussion regarding the psychiatric history. Efforts to gather information regarding psychiatric symptoms and background history were met with dismissal as irrelevant. McWilliams (1994) further notes that psychotic individuals have a marked incapacity to stand aside from their psychological problems and regard them dispassionately. M believed she suffered at the hands of other's social ignorance of her transgender status, and that her mental illness and all of its ramifications reflected this same ignorance. It became clear that a suitable setting in the public sector would have to include a resource for understanding and supporting M's transgender concerns, or a significant barrier in managing her mental illness would remain. An affirmative transgender environment seemed requisite if she was to differentiate the psychological impact of her transgender status from that of her mental illness.

The therapeutic process was significantly influenced by the initial telephone interview and multiple telephone interactions. These contacts led to identification of specific signs and symptoms of M's psychiatric illness, and revealed much about M's character formation, adaptive capacities, and defensive organization. What subsequently emerged in the course of treatment was a meaningful explanation of how M's early experiences were accounted for in her character and adult behaviors.

The student therapist's prior training experiences had required him to explain the patient's symptoms along with diagnostic impressions discussed in supervision after two or three intake evaluations. In M's case, however, this process would have reinforced her tendency to feel misunderstood, and would have led to a misunderstanding of the structure of her personality and how it developed. For instance, the disclosure of her name selection occurred after one year into the course of treatment. Her initial denial of having served in the military was later repudiated when she disclosed the Marine Corps discharge in the context of her first psychiatric hospitalization. Developing flexibility with this process through supervision created the opportunity to collaboratively learn how M ordered the events of her life, and created an environment for M to disclose and explore the meaning of long held beliefs regarding victimization and entitlement to compensation and relief.

M's denial of mental illness was remarkable. Her discourse on being misdiagnosed and mistreated raised fears in an inexperienced student therapist that he too would fail her just as all the others had. But, understanding M's defenses against accepting her mental illness clarified how an understanding of her denial and confusion would be a critical goal in the therapy. This further reinforced the notion that it would be necessary to differentiate her transgender issues from major mental illness, and to understand how the two interacted.

M articulated the details of prior hospitalizations, depressive symptoms, psychotic experiences, and the need for medication to prevent future decompensations. She spoke of her feelings regarding homelessness and loss. Attempts to explore these experiences were met with either minimizing their impact, or even refusal to accept that they actually happened. The therapist feared that exploration in this area would cause a rupture in the alliance.

Reflection and interpretation of M's subjective experience towards the therapist, while not completely recognized by M, was therapeutically effective, and created a change in the course of the treatment. These transferential issues were important in understanding M as a person, and not simply as someone with symptoms requiring management. Although M had not accepted her schizophrenia diagnosis, she became more interactive, spontaneous, and curious as to the meaning of her experiences.

Possibly the most difficult area in M's treatment was understanding her identification as a male-to-female transgender person. Her understanding appeared concrete and immature, incomplete in some meaningful way. M reported feeling different and socially uncomfortable from a very early age. She reported being harassed as a child for being effeminate. She enjoyed dressing in her sister's clothing until caught, a seminal event of intense interpersonal humiliation. She hid behind a male facade until her thirties, and wrestled with the confusion of whether she was gay. She talked of what it was like to be observed by others, with fears that were realized when she became the victim of the physical attack while in female attire. She spoke of her male and female identities as discreet, but not dissociated entities. Attempts to help M reconcile her identity were met with resistance.

The case of M raised concerns regarding the appropriateness of clinical work at the student level of training with patients who identify as transgender and suffer from major mental illness. Supervision provided an opportunity to explore and determine how to best serve M, and clarified ways to integrate personal experience into the therapy. The content provided by M in her narrative seemed less challenging than whether *Mark* or *Maria* provided it. M's "double-stigma" also functioned on multiple levels. The complications of her gender status, and the social and interpersonal difficulties associated with mental illness, created a complex, overlapping duality which became an important focus in her sessions (see Table 1, for a summary). Rarely were the two topics discussed in a single session, and attempts to link them were often dismissed. Furthermore, *Mark* focused on symptoms of mental illness, while *Maria* focused on transgender issues.

When the therapist's anxiety regarding the disparity between M's transgender and mental illness concerns was confronted, a primary goal of treatment emerged. M wanted to be understood by others, and this appeared to be a projection of her need to understand herself. The confusion and anxiety that this triggered for her therapist came from an identification with that projection. M had provided a glimpse into the subjective experience of her life, and her need to be viewed and understood as a person, rather than as an aggregate of symptoms, and the target of the humiliation and disrespect that is so common for the transgendered person.

The need for residential placement is widespread among those with serious mental illness in the public sector, and with M, this became a source of significant clinical concern that subsumed issues of gender and religion. The phenomenology of her transgender identity changed during her course of treatment, after being re-contextualized in her living situation. This created yet another challenge in the continuity of her care. She received services from a Christian residential apartment program, and each of three residential counselors during the course of treatment had an influence on her gender identity. She began to live full-time as a woman, while working with a supportive and accepting residential counselor of six years. According to M, her second counselor, assigned eight months into her present treatment setting, had strong Christian fundamentalist beliefs, denounced her transgender status, and encouraged her to reject her transgender identity for religious reasons. It was never clear whether M's perception of this counselor was accurate, or whether this counselor may have tried to encourage M to postpone addressing the stressful transgender concerns until she was more stable psychiatrically. Four months later, M was assigned a new counselor and she returned to her female identity, but was unable to live as a woman, having donated her clothes to charity. For the therapist, this experience brought home the need for sufficient corroboration and case management in addition to dyadic and group therapy.

Distinguishing gender identity disorder from schizophrenia, and the possibility as to whether the two can independently coexist, is a subject that continues to be actively debated (Campo et al., 2003). The *DSM-IV* (American Psychiatric Association, 1994) notes that having delusions of being a member of the opposite sex is quite rare. In the case of M, cross-gender identification was a stable, life-long trait that was present independent of psychotic decompensations and treatment (Table 1).

Zucker and Bradley (1995) report that on average, children with gender identity disorder (GID) appear to show as much general psychopathology as is shown by other children referred for clinical problems. Further, they state that there appears to be support for clinical observations that internalizing psychopathology is overrepresented among boys with GID. Zucker and Bradley conclude that multiple factors, including social ostracism and familial risk variables appear to account for the associated psychopathology, but that evidence regarding the causal role played by this pathology in the development of gender identity disorder is inconclusive. Several intimate biographical accounts of transgender individuals tell of the common personal turmoil that is experienced in response to the challenges they face (Bornstein, 1994; Feinberg, 1996; Wilchins, 1997; also see Leli and Drescher, 2004), providing some additional perspective for the clinician.

Standards of care for people with pervasive and persistent core gender concerns exist to guide clinicians in helping patients resolve the struggle with

TABLE 1. Categorization Based on M's Presentation

M's signs and symptoms of major mental illness	M as trangendered	Overlap between transgender status and mental illness
–Delusional perceptions –Auditory hallucinations –Compulsive writing –Functionally disabled when decompensated	–Early history typical of transgendered individuals: • early conviction of being female • not wanting penis • early effeminate behavior • few male friends –Cross-dressing independent of psychiatric decompensations –Efforts to "pass" as female independent of decompensations	–Episodic depressed mood –Suicide attempts –Stigma with isolation and rejection –Harassment –Social anxiety –Symptoms following assault: • withdrawal • mutism • anhedonia • vegetative symptoms • selective memory deficit

their gender identity issues (Harry Benjamin International Gender Dysphoria Association, 2001). Any psychiatric therapist working with individuals who have core gender identity concerns should familiarize themselves with these guidelines. M was already receiving cross-sex hormonal treatment from a public health clinic that specialized in LGBT medical treatment at the time of referral to the community mental health center. The medical clinic had previously determined that M met eligibility criteria for hormone therapy in adults. The essential need to collaborate with other agencies and clinicians involved in the treatment of a person undergoing gender transition was another unique aspect of this case.

Murphy, Rawlings and Howe (2002) state that the LGB[T] population reports a higher than average rate of therapy usage, including use of public psychiatric facilities, and that LGBT individuals share specific mental health concerns, including the fear of verbal and physical harassment if one's sexual or gender orientation is revealed. When coupled with a diagnosis of major mental illness, the challenging and unique hardships that can be a pervasive reality for such individuals came to be appreciated in a very direct way by this therapist.

Few programs exist that address "gay" concerns. Fewer still provide services for the transgendered individual. Many who identify as transgendered are more likely to be pathologized and ostracized. Such individuals risk loss of social and financial supports, leaving the public psychiatric sector as the only resource when they cannot afford private treatment. The transgender population in the public sector is less likely to afford sex reassignment surgery for economic reasons, as well. In the case presented here, the patient could not even afford clothing. Transgendered persons in the public sector are, therefore, less likely to realize an existence that is congruent anatomically and materially with their psychological identity, creating a life-long struggle for acceptance that adds to the existent stigmas which they face as transgendered individuals and persons suffering from major mental illness.

Working with M provided a formidable clinical learning experience, one that is not usually available in an academic setting. Based on the experience with this case, it is probably not unreasonable to propose that transgender individuals who present in the public sector are more likely to face significant psychosocial and economic difficulties that can be particularly challenging. This case afforded the therapist an opportunity to understand and usefully address the relative contribution of many factors and their interactions, and to experience and balance uncertainty in therapy sessions, while providing support, protection, education, and the invaluable occasion to explore and work towards resolution of the many issues that create so many barriers for these individuals.

REFERENCES

American Psychiatric Association (1994), *Diagnostic and Statistical Manual of Mental Disorders, Fourth Edition*. Washington, DC: American Psychiatric Press.

Bornstein, K. (1994), *Gender Outlaw: On Men, Women and the Rest of Us*. New York: Vintage Books.

Campo, J., Nijman, H., Merckelbach, H. & Evers, C. (2003), Psychiatric comorbidity of gender identity disorders: A survey among Dutch psychiatrists. *American J. Psychiatry,* 160(7):1332-1336.

Feinberg, L. (1996), *Transgender Warriors: Making History from Joan of Arc to Dennis Rodman*. Boston: Beacon Press.

Harry Benjamin International Gender Dysphoria Association (2001), *The Harry Benjamin International Gender Dysphoria Association's Standards of Care for Gender Identity Disorders, Sixth Version*. HBIGDA Website (*http://www.hbigda.org/socv6sm.pdf*).

Leli, U. & Drescher, J. (2004), *Transgender Subjectivities: A Clinician's Guide*. New York: Haworth Press.

McWilliams, N. (1994), *Psychoanalytic Diagnosis; Understanding Personality Structure in Clinical Practice.* New York: The Guilford Press.

Murphy, J.A., Rawlings, E.I. & Howe, S.R. (2002), A survey of clinical psychologists on treating lesbian, gay, and bisexual clients. *Professional Psychology: Research and Practice*, 33:183-189.

Wilchins, R. A. (1997), *Read My Lips: Sexual Subversion and the End of Gender.* Ithaca, NY: Firebrand Books.

Zucker, K.J. & Bradley, S.M. (1995), *Gender Identity Disorder and Psychosexual Problems in Children and Adolescents.* New York: The Guilford Press.

An Interview
with Francis G. Lu, MD

Ronald E. Hellman, MD

Francis G. Lu, MD, is Professor of Clinical Psychiatry, University of California, San Francisco (UCSF). He is also the Director of the Cultural Competence and Diversity Program, Department of Psychiatry at San Francisco General Hospital, where he has worked for over 26 years.

Dr. Lu received his medical degree from Dartmouth Medical School and completed residency training at Mount Sinai Medical Center, New York. He is the founder of the Asian/Pacific American Psychiatric Inpatient Program, which served as a model for 5 other programs serving Black, Latino, women, gay/lesbian and HIV patients. In 1987, the American Psychiatric Association (APA) awarded these programs a Certificate of Significant Achievement. In 1999, the American College of Psychiatrists awarded the Creativity in Psychiatric Education Award to these programs.

As a Distinguished Fellow of the APA, Dr. Lu has contributed to the areas of cultural psychiatry; psychiatric education; film and the transpersonal; and the interface of psychiatry and religion/spirituality through his presentations and more than 40 publications. He has participated on expert panels and advisory committees for cultural competence service and training projects sponsored by the American Psychiatric Association, the Office of the Surgeon General, DHHS Office of Minority Health, SAMHSA Center for Mental

Ronald E. Hellman is Program Director for the LesBiGay & Transgender Affirmative Program, South Beach Psychiatric Center, 25 Flatbush Avenue, 3rd Floor, Brooklyn, NY 11217 (E-mail: SBOPREH@gw.omh.state.ny.us).

[Haworth co-indexing entry note]: "An Interview with Francis G. Lu, MD." Hellman, Ronald E. Co-published simultaneously in *Journal of Gay & Lesbian Psychotherapy* (The Haworth Medical Press, an imprint of The Haworth Press, Inc.) Vol. 8, No. 3/4, 2004, pp. 143-154; and: *Handbook of LGBT Issues in Community Mental Health* (ed: Ronald E. Hellman, and Jack Drescher) The Haworth Medical Press, an imprint of The Haworth Press, Inc., 2004, pp. 143-154. Single or multiple copies of this article are available for a fee from The Haworth Document Delivery Service [1-800-HAWORTH, 9:00 a.m. - 5:00 p.m. (EST). E-mail address: docdelivery@haworthpress.com].

Health Services, the California Endowment and the Templeton Foundation. He currently serves on the California State Department of Mental Health Cultural Competence Advisory Committee and the UCSF Chancellor's Advisory Committee on Diversity.

The APA awarded him the 2001 Kun-Po Soo Award for his work in integrating Asian issues into psychiatry; in 2002, he received a Special APA Presidential Commendation for his work in cross-cultural psychiatry. Dr. Lu currently chairs the APA Council on Minority Mental Health and Health Disparities. In 2002, the National Alliance for the Mentally Ill awarded him an Exemplary Psychiatrist Award for exceptional cultural awareness and sensitivity. Also in 2002, he served as Executive Scientific Advisor for a 58-minute training videotape "The Culture of Emotions" about the *DSM-IV* Outline for Cultural Formulation. In 2003, the Association of Gay and Lesbian Psychiatrists (AGLP), the parent organization of the *Journal of Gay & Lesbian Psychotherapy*, awarded him its Distinguished Service Award. He is a Fellow of the Pacific Rim College of Psychiatrists and a Member of the American College of Psychiatrists and the Group for the Advancement of Psychiatry, Cultural Psychiatry Committee. Since 1987, Dr. Lu has co-led 17 five-day film seminars at Esalen Institute in Big Sur, CA exploring film and the transpersonal.

JGLP: You were honored in May, 2003 with an award by AGLP at the Annual Meeting of the American Psychiatric Association in San Francisco. Can you tell us about the award and the work you did to be recognized by AGLP?

Dr. Lu: I was extremely humbled to be honored with this award. I understand that I am the first non-gay psychiatrist to have received it, and I am very grateful to the Association for thinking of me. I believe that the award came about for my work on several fronts in the areas of cultural competence and diversity. First of all, at the service level, designing our ethnic minority focus inpatient programs at San Francisco General Hospital, which I can speak about in a moment. Secondly, the advancements in curriculum in psychiatry residency training concerning the accreditation standards, both in the 1995 and 2001 versions. Thirdly, in my work that has been recognized by the APA at the Annual Meeting in 2002. I received a Special Presidential Commendation from the APA President, Richard Harding, for my cross-cultural psychiatry work. Lastly, I have chaired the Council on Minority Mental Health and Health Disparities of the APA since 2002. The Committee on Gay, Lesbian, and Bisexual Concerns reports to that council.

JGLP: How did you become involved in cultural psychiatry?

Dr. Lu: I completed my residency at Mt. Sinai Hospital in New York City in 1977, but I did not receive any training there in cross-cultural or minority issues. I was attracted to the idea of returning to California, where I was born in 1949, to be in a more culturally diverse environment. In 1979, I attended two conferences sponsored by the National Institute for Mental Health to create training curricula for Asian-American issues in the realm of psychiatry. I was one of four Asian-American psychiatrists selected to participate in this effort. On my way back from that meeting in Chicago, I thought it would be very interesting to create a focus inpatient unit at San Francisco General Hospital (SFGH) on Asian issues. I was the Unit Chief at that time.

This made sense for San Francisco, because 21% of the city's population was Asian, and a large number of Asians came to the hospital. SFGH was the only public hospital in San Francisco. Also, at SFGH, we did have outpatient and day treatment programs that focused on Asian patients. So I thought it made sense to create an inpatient unit to complement those services to provide a comprehensive system of care for those patients. Around the same time, President Carter's Commission on Mental Health created a section on Asian issues, and they recommended the concept of developing teams that could cross catchment areas for service provision, so as to maximize the impact of scarce human resources, and to increase visibility of such services.

The Asian Focus Unit was initiated in 1980, and subsequent to that, we developed, over many years, focused programs involving other ethnic minority groups at SFGH. I have been very involved with the development of these services, as well as resident recruitment and mentorship at the University of California at San Francisco (UCSF). I have been on the Residency Selection Committee for more than 18 years. So, that is how it began.

JGLP: You started with the Asian Unit and then expanded?

Dr. Lu: There are actually five inpatient units altogether. The Asian unit, a Black focus unit, a Latino and Women's focus unit, and the Lesbian/Gay/Bisexual/Transgender and HIV focus unit. The fifth one is a Forensic unit that provides short term inpatient care for people in the prison system.

I should reiterate a point that is important to understand. First of all, these are focus units, rather than a form of segregation or apartheid. We have patients and staff of all ethnicities and sexual orientations on all of the units. However, the units are meant to provide some focus of expertise, so that when there are patients who come to the hospital that might benefit from such specialized services, those services will be available.

For example, on the Asian focus unit, we have about 14 Asian languages and dialects of Chinese spoken by the staff, language being one of the obvious characteristics that might be important to a patient if they have limited English proficiency. There are also cultural issues that patients might have that would be important to recognize, understand, and work with while they are on the unit.

JGLP: What has been the response of heterosexual, Caucasian patients? Are they distributed among the focus units?

Dr. Lu: Yes, these patients are treated in the various focus units. Some patients have raised the question of why we do not have a unit for them. We do not really have a good answer. I would say that what may be acceptable here in San Francisco may seem rather radical, out of place, or be completely unworkable in another location. The focus units are unique–this is the only place in the country where we have this kind of clustering, although there are isolated focus units elsewhere, including New York City.

This works in San Francisco because of a number of factors. First, there are the demographics of the population here, which is less than 50% Caucasian. Currently, about a third of the City is Asian, about 14% Latino, 8% Black, and about 15% estimated to be lesbian, gay, bisexual, or transgender. Second, these minority groups tend to over-utilize the services of the public hospital relative to their population. Third, since the 1970s in San Francisco, we have had outpatient services that also have a similar focus, so there is a very strong tradition to provide these kinds of services here. The inpatient units are an extension of that tradition, and are consistent with this particular form of service provision.

Currently, the Director of our Community Behavioral Health Services is Bob Cabaj, MD. He, of course, has been a wonderful leader on gay and lesbian issues for many years. He has been quite supportive of this kind of focus structure, as well. I think it is important for your readers to understand that this may not work everywhere. I think everyone knows that San Francisco is a little different than other parts of the country.

JGLP: When you have a patient that might identify with more than one unit, say a gay, Asian patient, do they get to choose the unit they would prefer?

Dr. Lu: Yes. We try as much as much as possible to ask about patient preferences. Sometimes, when patients are in the emergency room, where they may be quite psychotic or unable to process that information for other reasons, the clinician may need to make a decision based on fragmentary information. Patients that are admitted to a particular unit can later be transferred to another if that would be helpful or desirable. I think the important thing is always the individual patient, and trying to understand what the particular and relevant needs are regarding that specific person at that time.

For example, a gay, Asian patient might have issues much more related to sexual orientation than ethnicity. Gene Nakajima and Kewchang Lee have written about how multiple cultural factors can be very intertwined and hard to sort out.[1] There may be a particular relevance of one set of issues rather than another. Obviously, if a gay, Asian patient speaks Cantonese, it might make more sense to have that patient on the Asian unit where our Cantonese speaking staff are located.

JGLP: Have your programs developed according to your expectations, or have they evolved in ways that were unanticipated?

Dr. Lu: When we started, we had three goals: services, training, and research. I think we have done fairly well on the first two, but the research area is not as developed as we had wanted 20 years ago. In reality, working on acute inpatient services, especially here at SFGH, is very hard and demanding. Sometimes, it is quite difficult to recruit and retain psychiatrists to work here. I think our focus programs actually help with that recruitment and retention, in that we are able to find people who find working on the focus units particularly interesting and meaningful. However, sometimes that is a double-edged sword, because we try to find people with specialized skills, and they can be in great demand when there is a low supply. So, it is always a challenge to recruit and retain attending psychiatrists.

In terms of training, our focus units have been a positive source of interest among the resident applicants. They generally come with some interest in these units, recognizing that they are unique. I think their existence has encouraged our recruitment of residents, both those of ethnic minority and those not of ethnic minority who are interested in cultural issues. In these two respects, I think we have made considerable progress.

JGLP: What have been some of the advantages and disadvantages of working in the public sector?

Dr. Lu: Beauty is in the eyes of the beholder. What I mean is that this kind of work really calls for a match between the setting, the psychiatrist, and the other staff. I think the reason many of us stay on is the "calling," if you will, to work with the underserved, people that would not normally be getting quality services. Especially here in San Francisco, with SFGH being the only acute, public hospital, there is special meaning associated with working here. This hospital was created in the 1860s, so it is a place with some history. We are also a major teaching hospital for UCSF, with a relationship going back to the 1880s. This is a feature of our service that faculty find very attractive, as we have the ability to recruit, supervise, and work with excellent medical students and residents to whom we pass on the legacy. As one grows older, I think one thinks more about the issue of legacy and passing the torch from one generation to the next. In this department, where the focus has been on cultural issues, I think that has meant a lot to many people here, and brings them here, as well.

I think the disadvantages or difficulties are endemic to the public sector today, especially with our financial crises at all levels. Considering the constant budget deliberations and reductions or possible reductions, our department has done quite well in staving off major cutbacks through the years. We have been quite fortunate in San Francisco, but I am sure in other parts of the country, it has been quite different.

JGLP: I understand that your efforts helped to save the focus units from budget cuts several years ago.

Dr. Lu: Yes, that was a very interesting experience. This was in the year 2000. The City was having the usual budget deficit problems and one proposal from the Director of Public Health was to eliminate one of our inpatient units. Our department, instead of simply agreeing to that, came together and mounted an effort to save one of our inpatient units. We hired a lobbyist, put out a media campaign, had press conferences that supervisors (City legislative council members) attended, had meetings with supervisors and their aides, met with editorial boards of the two daily newspapers here, wrote letters to the editor, garnered the support of organizations like the Police Officers Association, and eventually saved the unit.

I visited City Hall more times in those three months than in all of the previous years I had been in San Francisco. I felt very compelled to work along these lines. I felt there was a special calling to protect one of our inpatient units. It was really a departmental effort. Our Chair was behind these efforts, with some political risk to him. We even funded the effort on our own through contributions from the Department. It was quite an experience.

JGLP: How has the political climate affected the viability of programs like this?

Dr. Lu: This past budget year was the worst that I have seen in San Francisco in 25 years. Many mental health programs were on the chopping block. They did not target our focus units. In the end, much of the funding was restored, but some was not. I think it is a major problem, and this is reflected, for example, in the recently released President's Commission on Mental Health report under President Bush.[2] This came out in July, 2003 and diagnosed the situation fairly accurately regarding the tremendous gaps we have in mental health care. The report enunciated six goals to close that gap. However, the Commission was told to be revenue neutral in coming up with solutions, so it left something to be desired.

The macro funding issue is also an enormous concern in terms of public mental health services in general. My hope is that we can encourage, in some way, people to do research in these areas to show that culturally competent services can reduce mental health disparities and be cost effective. It seems intuitively correct, but we desperately need evidence. We talk about evidence-based medicine now, and we urgently need research to substantiate that hypothesis.

JGLP: Are there other issues in addition to the budgetary concerns? For example, the influence of those in the Bush administration with conservative views, particularly around LGBT issues, who argue against the promotion of a "gay agenda." Has this type of conservative perspective affected the ability to maintain your LGBT program?

Dr. Lu: Here in San Francisco, there continues to be general support in that area. I am not aware of any cutbacks targeting our LGBT programs. However, I speak from a very privileged position here in San Francisco. In other parts of the country, such services may not even exist, or thoughts of developing such services might bring up resistance, or targeted cutbacks if they do exist. I would be interested to know what it is like in other parts of the country.

JGLP: The public sector typically serves those of lower socioeconomic status, and those with more severe disorders where insurance may not cover the total care needed. However, because you have this unique, specialized LGBT unit, has there been interest by those who would otherwise seek care in the private sector? Is this service available in the private sector?

Dr. Lu: It is not available in the private sector here in San Francisco. We have had some discussions with other agencies, such as Kaiser and other community mental health programs in surrounding counties, to reach agreement. If they have patients who might benefit from our focus units, they could be admitted and treated here at SFGH for some negotiated rate. However, we have not vigorously pursued those possibilities. We are in the public sector, and our first responsibility is to take care of those patients who might obtain services with great difficulty because they have no insurance, or they have MediCal (Medicaid), which is only accepted by a handful of hospitals on an inpatient basis. So, we have very few patients here hospitalized with private insurance.

JGLP: Is MediCal the primary source of funding for your services?

Dr. Lu: Yes. MediCal and Medicare reimbursements, which are partly federal and partly state funds, are the primary revenue sources. We also have general funds that come from the City to take care of the uninsured patients.

JGLP: What would your report card grade be for public psychiatry regarding the incorporation of culturally sensitive programming?

Dr. Lu: For the country overall, I would probably give it a "C." I think we have a long way to go. The glass is always half empty or half full. Although that is a truism, the older I get, the more I believe it. Let me give you some hopeful pointers. In March, 2003, the American College of Mental Health Administration had its annual meeting in Santa Fe.[3] The focus was on reducing mental health disparities. I was on a planning committee for that meeting, and had an excellent discussion about cultural competence and the goal of reducing mental health disparities.

Second, I believe that in the health field in general, there has been increasing concern about reducing health disparities. This started with President Clinton's presidential initiative in this area, and is also evident in the Surgeon General's 2001 *Report on Mental Health: Culture, Race, and Ethnicity.*[4] In the Bush Administration's July 2003 Presidential Commission Report, one of the six goals is eliminating mental health disparities.

Finally, in December, 2002, the Institute of Medicine issued a report entitled "Unequal Treatment: Confronting Racial and Ethnic Disparities in Health Care."[5] They clearly demonstrated that disparities exist for multifold reasons, including everything from clinician bias to systems issues. Now, the difficulty here, in terms of the LGBT perspective, is that a focus of many of these reports and initiatives has been on racial and ethnic differences, not so much on sexual orientation differences. However, I think the thrust on mental health disparities may be a useful one upon which the LGBT mental health community could focus, if it has not done so already, or to sharpen that focus. I think the focus on disparities is a very important lever to then say that culturally competent services might help reduce these disparities. This is an intuitive statement, a hypothesis that for which we need more evidence. However, I think it is a way of arguing for culturally competent services by giving a rationale that supports the need for LGBT services.

JGLP: Research in this area seems to be in its infancy?

Dr. Lu: Yes. I can speak in terms of racial and ethnic differences in the area of cultural competence. I am less familiar with the LGBT literature around disparities in health care. I know that some studies have been conducted, but in terms of bringing the literature together in a manner similar to the Institute of Medicine report, if such a report has not already been done, it could be extremely useful.

JGLP: What are your thoughts on using the leverage of re-licensure and re-accreditation to ensure that programs are culturally competent?

Dr. Lu: I am glad you brought that up. I think this is a very important area. For example, from the point of view of residency training programs in psychiatry, the 1995 accreditation standards did include, for the first time, mention of sexual orientation issues, along with ethnicity, race, gender, religious and spiritual issues. These were mandated to be included in the didactic curriculum of residency programs. How that gets interpreted by an accreditation team when they visit a program remains to be clearly understood and determined. In any case, that standard is now there.

In the 2001 standards, there were further modifications that continued the line of thinking that social and cultural issues were important in a number of different ways. For example, in case conferences, as related to diagnosis and treatment planning, the phenomenological, psychological, and neurobiological, as well as the social and cultural issues should be brought together as part of an integrative case formulation.

In terms of accreditation of programs, some very interesting developments have occurred over the last four or five years involving the Joint Commission on Accreditation of Healthcare Organizations (JCAHO) standards for spirituality. Again, how this is interpreted by individual programs remains to be seen, but at least there seems to be some attention being paid to this issue. I am not clear to what extent sexual orientation issues are mentioned in the JCAHO standards. But, if they are not there, then pointing out that the disparities exist and that it would, therefore, be important to attend to these issues, would be a way of getting this issue attention regarding general standards of care.

JGLP: Regarding education and training, has there been any effort to incorporate sexual minority issues in the evaluations for Board certification?

Dr. Lu: That is a very good question. I do not know, in terms of the Part I examination, to what extent questions around sexual and gender orientation are included. The problem with Part II in regards to social/cultural issues in general, is that, even though there is an expectation that psychosocial history, and so forth, be part of the comprehensive examination, typically in the 30 minutes, there is relatively little that can be obtained and discussed, and the focus tends to be on the differential diagnosis and treatment planning. That would certainly bear further assessment and advocacy.

JGLP: Who were some of the people that influenced your thinking in the area of cultural psychiatry?

Dr. Lu: I owe a great deal to the Group for the Advancement of Psychiatry and its Cultural Psychiatry Committee, of which I have been a member since 1993. People in that group include Ron Wintrob, Ezra Griffith from Yale, Pedro Ruiz, Renato Alarçon, Irma Bland, who just passed away in July 2003, and Joe

Yamamoto from UCLA, who recently retired. There are others in that group as well.

Second, there is the legacy of Asian American psychiatrists, who came before me. People like Luke Kim from UC Davis, Normund Wong, who was the President of AADPRT back in the 1980s. Another person is Evelyn Lee, who was a social worker and had a Doctorate of Education. She was a most important influence. She worked with me at SFGH from 1982 until 1990, where we co-led the Asian inpatient focus unit. She then moved on to become the executive director of RAMS, a community-based, non-profit mental health organization in San Francisco, from 1990 to 2003. She was a pioneering spirit, very enthusiastic about these issues, very politically savvy, clinically sharp, and administratively a brilliant woman, who unfortunately passed away suddenly in March, 2003 at age 58 of a heart attack. I'm sure I am leaving others out, but this would be a good start.

JGLP: Finally, do you have any insights or lessons for others about what you have learned over the years in developing and administrating culturally sensitive programming in the public sector?

Dr. Lu: First of all, it is terribly important to network at many levels. One is obviously the local level, to be, for example, part of a cultural competency and diversity committee within a department or organization in order to get a group together, have these concerns sanctioned by the authorities that be, and provide recommendations to the head of the organization or chief of the department concerning cultural competence and diversity. This would be a good way to begin to generate interest in this area. Sharing the burdens and tasks this way is also easier. And with that in mind, you could begin to look at services and training, and perhaps research efforts.

Second, to keep a broad focus that includes not only race and ethnicity, but sexual and gender orientation, class, as well as religious and spiritual issues. This is very important in preventing stereotyping, and underlies the complexity with which we are dealing.

Third, would be networking nationally. There are organizations where one can receive support, encouragement and inspiration, as well as very useful information. One would be the Society for the Study of Psychiatry and Culture. This group has an annual meeting in the fall every year. The Institute for Psychiatric Services of the APA is a useful meeting. A group known as the American Association of Community Psychiatrists is very active and presents at that meeting. This is a group that is very focused on working in the public sector.

The last thing to keep in mind is in the *I Ching*. It says, "perseverance furthers." I am celebrating 26 years at SFGH. Looking back, the institution has changed over time, I think in a generally positive direction, even though, on a day to day basis, it may seem pretty daunting and challenging. However, through all of that, it is always important to keep the bigger picture in mind.

NOTES

1. Nakajima, G., Chan, Y. & Lee, K. (1996), Mental health issues for gay and lesbian Asian Americans. In: *Textbook of Homosexuality and Mental Health*, eds. R. P. Cabaj and T. S. Stein. Washington, DC: American Psychiatric Press, pp. 563-582.

2. President's New Freedom Commission on Mental Health (2003), *Report on Mental Health*. Washington, DC: U.S. Government Printing Office.

3. Dougherty, R., ed. (2003), Executive summary of the March, 2003 summit, *Reducing Disparity: Achieving Equity in Behavioral Health Services*, American College of Mental Health Administration.

4. U.S. Department of Health and Human Services (2001), Mental health: Culture, race and ethnicity, In: *Mental Health: A Report of the Surgeon General*. Rockville, MD: U.S. Department of Health and Human Services, Public Health Service.

5. Smedley, B.D., Stith, A.Y. & Nelson, A.R., eds. (2002), Committee on Understanding and Eliminating Racial and Ethnic Disparities in Health Care, *Unequal Treatment: Confronting Racial and Ethnic Disparities in Health*. Washington, DC: National Academy Press.

SELECTED BIBLIOGRAPHY

Group for the Advancement of Psychiatry, Cultural Psychiatry Committee (1996), *Alcoholism in the United States: Racial and Ethnic Considerations*. Washington, DC: American Psychiatric Press.

Larson, D., Lu, F. & Sawyers, J., eds. (1997), *Model Curriculum for Psychiatry Residency Training Programs: Religion and Spirituality in Clinical Practice (Revised Edition)*. Rockville, MD: National Institute for Healthcare Research.

Association of American Medical Colleges (1999), Task force report on spirituality, cultural issues and end of life care. In: *Medical School Objectives Report, Report III*. Washington, DC: Association of American Medical Colleges.

Gee, K., Du, N., Akiyama, K. & Lu, F. (1999), The Asian Focus Unit at UCSF: An 18-year perspective. In: *Cross Cultural Psychiatry*, eds. J. Herrera, W. Lawson & J. Sramek. New York: Wiley, 275-285.

Lu, F., Lee, K. & Prathikanti, S. (1999), Minorities in academic psychiatry. In: *Handbook of Psychiatric Education and Faculty Development*, ed. J. Kay. Washington, DC: American Psychiatric Press, 109-124.

Lu, F. (2000), Religious and spiritual issues in psychiatric residency education and training. In: *Religion and Psychiatry*, ed. J. Boehnlein. Washington, DC: American Psychiatric Press, 159-168.

Spurlock, J., Munoz, R., Thompson, J. & Lu, F. (2000), Minorities in American psychiatry. In: *American Psychiatry Since World War II*, eds. R. Menninger & J. Nemiah. Washington, DC: American Psychiatric Press, 594-611.

Lu, F. (2001), Appendix B: Annotated bibliography on cultural psychiatry and related topics. In: *Concise Guide to Cultural Psychiatry*, ed. A. Gaw. Washington, DC: American Psychiatric Press, 205-212.

Group for the Advancement of Psychiatry, Cultural Psychiatry Committee (2002), *Cultural Assessment in Clinical Psychiatry*. Washington, DC: American Psychiatric Press.

Lu, F. (2002), Executive Scientific Advisor, *The Culture of Emotions: A Cultural Competency and Diversity Training Program*. Videotape. Boston: Fanlight Productions.

Lu, F., Du, N., Gaw, A. & Lin, K.-M. (2002), A Curriculum for learning about Asian-American patients in psychiatric residencies. *Academic Psychiatry*, 26(4): 225-236.

Lu., F. (2003), A Silver Anniversary for an Asian American Academic Psychiatrist. *Academic Psychiatry*, 27(3): 206-207.

Interview with
Barbara E. Warren, PsyD, CASAC, CPP

Ronald E. Hellman, MD

Before her recent promotion to initiate a new department for the Lesbian, Gay, Bisexual and Transgender (LGBT) Community Center of New York City, Barbara E. Warren PsyD, CASAC, CPP was the Center's Director of Mental Health and Social Services. A faculty member of the New York State Academy of Addiction Studies, she was the principal author of the first official state-sponsored training curriculum addressing sensitivity to LGBT clients.[1] She has taught in the graduate programs of Fordham University, Hunter College, Yeshiva University and Columbia University; has developed and taught courses for alcohol and drug counselors, both locally and nationally; and provides diversity training to human services organizations and treatment facilities.

Dr. Warren holds a doctorate in counseling psychology from the Florida Institute of Technology's School of Psychology and is a credentialed alcoholism and substance abuse counselor and substance abuse prevention professional in New York State. She has 25 years of experience in the development and implementation of mental health, substance abuse and social service programs in community based settings. In 1988, she was hired as the founding director of the Center's Project Connect, one of the first LGBT-identified alcohol and drug abuse prevention and intervention programs in the country. Under Dr.

Ronald E. Hellman is Program Director for the LesBiGay & Transgender Affirmative Program, South Beach Psychiatric Center, 25 Flatbush Avenue, 3rd Floor, Brooklyn, NY 11217 (E-mail: SBOPREH@gw.omh.state.ny.us).

[Haworth co-indexing entry note]: "Interview with Barbara E. Warren, PsyD, CASAC, CPP." Hellman, Ronald E. Co-published simultaneously in *Journal of Gay & Lesbian Psychotherapy* (The Haworth Medical Press, an imprint of The Haworth Press, Inc.) Vol. 8, No. 3/4, 2004, pp. 155-170; and: *Handbook of LGBT Issues in Community Mental Health* (ed: Ronald E. Hellman, and Jack Drescher) The Haworth Medical Press, an imprint of The Haworth Press, Inc., 2004, pp. 155-170. Single or multiple copies of this article are available for a fee from The Haworth Document Delivery Service [1-800-HAWORTH, 9:00 a.m. - 5:00 p.m. (EST). E-mail address: docdelivery@haworthpress.com].

Warren's direction, the Center developed a comprehensive mental health and social services department providing a continuum of substance abuse and other counseling, advocacy, referral and training services to LGBT adults and youth from diverse backgrounds. In 1996, Dr. Warren developed and implemented the Center's first smoking intervention program, Becoming Smoke Free With Pride, which today is the Center's LGBT Smoke Free Project, providing prevention, cessation and advocacy.

In addition to her work in the area of direct services, Dr. Warren has also represented the Center and the needs of the LGBT communities in an advocacy and policy capacity. Working closely with Carmen Vazquez, the Center's Director of Public Policy, Dr. Warren has been active in funding and policy initiatives of the New York State Network of Lesbian, Gay, Bisexual and Transgender Health and Human Services Providers and the National Association of Lesbian and Gay Community Centers. As a consultant on policy and program development, she has worked with numerous city, state and federal agencies, including the New York State Department of Health, the New York State Office of Alcoholism and Substance Abuse Services, the Federal Centers for Substance Abuse Prevention and Substance Abuse Treatment and, as the first Community Co-Chair of New York City's HIV Prevention Planning Group, with the Federal Centers for Disease Control and Prevention.

As part of her special interest in working with the transgender communities, in 1990 Dr. Warren initiated the development of the Center's peer empowerment program for transgender and transsexual people, the Gender Identity Project, which has served as a model and a resource for transgender services worldwide. As a member of the Harry Benjamin International Gender Dysphoria Association, she has been an outspoken and powerful advocate both for the inclusion of transgender professionals in the organizational membership and structure of the Association, and for a consumer voice in the development of treatment standards and strategies. She is the author of several articles on community approaches to HIV prevention for the transgender communities and is a noted speaker and trainer in this area as well.

JGLP: You were recently appointed Director of Organization and Development at the LGBT Community Center in NYC after being its Director of Mental Health for many years. What do you do in your current position and how did your previous experience as Director of Mental Health prepare you?

Dr. Warren: The actual position has a long-winded title, which is Director of Organizational Development, Planning and Research. I am responsible for a number of things in that division, including new program development at the Center, both in terms of external program development, such as a new "Crystal Meth" project to do outreach and education with men who have sex with men who are abusing that drug or are at risk for abusing it. I am also responsible for helping the organization look at its needs and consider restructuring to better able do its work.

The research part focuses on our interventions involving mental health, social services, HIV support, emerging cultural programming, political work, and health promotion. We knew we were being effective, but we did not have the data to demonstrate this. We did not have any mechanism in place to evaluate this in a systematic way. So both to demonstrate to funders that we were being effective, and also to help the community look at innovative ways to work on health and related issues, we wanted to be able to objectively document outcomes and demonstrate what we were doing.

For example, one question we are trying to answer is whether it makes a difference to offer mental health services in a community center rather than a hospital or clinic. Is it more effective for an LGBT person to come into an LGBT identified setting? Or does it just have to be an effective intervention, and it does not really matter in what cultural context it occurs. Anecdotally, we think it does matter, but there is not a lot of research to demonstrate that. Yet, we are seeing that people seem to be more comfortable talking about certain concerns in an LGBT group setting, that they would be uncomfortable talking about in a mixed setting.

Another area of interest has to do with the different ways of transmitting prevention and treatment messages. In our program to help people quit smoking, for example, we have pioneered a "contemplator model" of intervention. Most smoking cessation groups are action-oriented groups. We are running a "Not-Quite-Ready-to-Quit" group for people who do not think they are ready to stop, but are thinking about it. It is a group for people who are not coming to the group to quit, but who are coming to figure out whether they want to quit. People in the cessation field are very interested in this type of group, and are looking to see if it is worth expanding this approach. We have some very early results based on only four or five such groups—with a total number of about 100 subjects—but we are already seeing some indications that the increase in motivation may be significant.

As the mental health door opened wider at the Center, I was already doing program development, fund raising, training, and policy related work, so it was natural for me to move into that position. I went from directing mental health and social services programs, and growing programs, for example, from a $100,000 alcoholism services budget, to a $2,000,000 multi-services budget. It became impossible for one person to manage all the operations of the programs and work on program development, research, and planning. It was necessary to create two positions, and so last year I was promoted to my current position and Eleanor Nealy, who had previously worked in a former position of mine, returned and was appointed to the Director of Mental Health position.

JGLP: When did you become the Director of Mental Health?

Dr. Warren: This is my sixteenth year at the Center. I was the original director for Project Connect, which began in 1987. This program provides assessment, short-term individual and couples counseling, and recovery support groups for LGBT persons having difficulty with alcohol and drugs. It also provides clinical referrals, psychoeducation, and clinical training. For those with HIV/ AIDS, it provides recovery-readiness counseling, relapse prevention interventions, and education addressing the link between drug use and HIV. This was the Center's first funded program from the New York State Division of Alcoholism and Alcohol Abuse, which is now the New York State Office of Alcoholism and Substance Abuse Services. By 1991, we had four programs that included Project Connect, Youth Enrichment Services, CenterBridge–an AIDS bereavement program, and the Gender Identity Project. In 1992, I was appointed Director of Mental Health and Social Services in order to direct the four programs.

JGLP: Where and how did your interest in this work originate?

Dr. Warren: I was a psychologist but started out in social work. I received a doctorate in counseling psychology and then worked for Pace University in the student counseling center. Pace, at that time, did not have a gay and lesbian student group. I was a very sympathetic ally when a number of gay students came to me, and I helped them start a group at Pace. One of the students was volunteering at the Community Health Project, which was housed in the Center, of which I had no knowledge at the time. He brought me a copy of an ad for a position at the Center. This gay student was quite encouraging, and thought I would be perfect working there. I had to laugh, because I am not gay-identified. As it turned out, I met with Richard Burns, the Executive Director at the Center. We knew some people in common from our days in Provincetown, and Richard seemed to like me. It was an important position that would entail implementing the Center's first grant. He offered me the job, but I was reluctant to take it because I thought it should really be someone who was gay or lesbian identified, as the position would have a lot of visibility. But Richard was persistent. He had this vision of bringing in someone who was a straight ally that could do the work, represent the gay community, but also reach out and represent the Center to the non-gay world. So, that is how it happened, and I am still here.

Over the years, one of the things I found so compelling about working on LGBT issues is how progressive the LGBT community has been in terms of cutting edge social justice issues. Many transgender people started coming to the Center, and many of those who are now leaders in the transgender community derived their support from those at the Center. So, we are very proud of the Center in this area.

JGLP: Who were the people that influenced your thinking in terms of your work in the public sector?

Dr. Warren: I would say that Richard Burns had a great deal of influence. He saw the potential for institutions like the Center a long time ago, particularly in terms of advocating for a bigger share of the public sector pie. He developed a strategy in which we coupled going after federal and municipal funding with our voter registration project. If you are going to have your hand out for tax dollars, you also have to able to document that you pay taxes. The voter registration and mobilization project that the Center embarked on began to get the message out that "we're here, we're queer," we vote, we pay taxes, and we deserve a fair share of funding for the needs of the LGBT community. As the years went on, he got me more interested in policy, and I got him more interested in psychology.

The other thing that happened was my getting involved with the Center at a time that coincided with the AIDS epidemic. Couple that with the opportunity to make LGBT health care issues more visible. The hard thing was that AIDS was clearly an important issue, but it was not the only health care issue in the community, and for a while, we had to fight the notion that the only need in the LGBT community was AIDS-related. Often, I would be involved in some funding or policy initiative, and there was this backlash effect. Funders would say that they had already dealt with AIDS, and I would have to educate them as to the range of health concerns that the LGBT community faced. The opposite has happened in the last two years. Fewer people are dying, and AIDS has faded a bit on the radar screen, so we have to remind people that this is still a major concern in the community.

I have spent a lot of time working with AIDS activists in a variety of capacities, from those working on the community level, to those in ACT UP, to those working in AIDS research. A big influence on me in terms of policy development was Richard Elovich at Gay Men's Health Crisis (GMHC) in the early 90s. He was an actor who became involved in AIDS policy work as a gay man in ACT UP, and ended up in the Policy Department at GMHC. We both had this "community chemistry" where we would hook up our ideas and energies, which resulted in many collaborative efforts between GMHC and the Center. For example, they were very focused on AIDS and HIV, but they were not that savvy about substance abuse and other mental health issues in the gay community that could contribute to the risk for HIV. The Center had a substance abuse program. Richard and I talked about the need to address the two issues in the same breath. At that time, most groups were either about substance abuse recovery or about HIV, but they were not necessarily addressed together. As the Center gained a reputation for its substance abuse program, we had straight people who were HIV positive and did not feel comfortable being out about being HIV positive in the heterosexual community, coming to the Center for help. This was because they knew we were recovery oriented and had experience working with those with HIV. This was in the late 1980s and early 90s, before it became more routine for mainstream agencies to address risk factors for HIV.

Then, in the mid-90s, Carmen Vasquez came to the Center as the Director of Public Policy. In the last ten years, she and I have worked closely together, and we have had the opportunity to create visibility and credibility regarding the Center's role in health care policy and service development. We have had the opportunity to go to Washington and work together, I think in a way that other, more nationally focused LGBT organizations were not doing. They were focused on legislation. Carmen and I were walking the halls in federal agencies, creating relationships with project officers on a very much more agency/community level. As a result, we were able to create access to policy makers and federal agencies in DC. We were able to get federal grants for the Center, and we put LGBT health care issues on the mental health policy and service radar screen in Washington. In addition to calling attention to the issues in Washington and Albany, we were doing collaborative community work, training local, mainstream agencies.

I have also worked with people at the community level, such as Rosalyne Blumenstein, who was the Center's first director of the Gender Identity Project. She was originally a program participant in the early 90s, quickly became a volunteer, then a student intern, counselor, then the director. People like Rosalyne not only had the courage to do the work professionally, but to be out publicly, which is really a tough thing. She would go out and do presentations in the community and say, "Hi, I'm a social worker and a woman of transsexual experience." That is not an easy thing to do.

JGLP: What are the mental health and social services that the Center has provided?

Dr. Warren: Our first program was Project Connect, the Center's alcohol and drug program, which provides individual, couples, and group counseling, smoking cessation groups, recovery readiness assessments, education, professional training, advocacy, and HIV prevention. Then we received a grant to start Youth Enrichment Services.

We grew from that to develop the Gender Identity Project, which provides individual peer counseling to the transgender community, support groups, information and links to medical and social service resources, drug counseling, HIV prevention and intervention services, forums, community education, professional training, and an annual transgender health empowerment conference.

In 1991, we started CenterBridge, our bereavement project. At that time, everyone was starting to talk about learning to live with AIDS, but nobody wanted to deal with dying from AIDS. In the late 1980s and early 90s, I was going to a funeral a week. Gay men were hit especially hard and there was a lot of grief in the community. But the political spin at that time was to emphasize living with AIDS, not dying from AIDS. The phrasing changed at that time from "people with AIDS" to "people living with AIDS." I can understand why people did that, but at the Center, we were seeing a lot of people who were secretly grieving, and some were drinking and drugging because of that, and also sero-converting. When we first started the program, no one wanted to fund it. Finally, the New York Community Trust gave us a small amount of money, and we were able to hire Dana Rose. He also created Ujima Community, which used Africological approaches to grief and loss resolution.

A structural change took place as the number of programs grew, and now the services are organized according to different functions. Last year, under Eleanor's leadership, we formally ended all the separate programs, and now we have a continuum of adult mental health and social services called CenterCare, which stands for Counseling, Advocacy, Recovery, and Education. The Youth Program still functions as a separate entity with a wide array of functions and services.

So, we started out as an alcohol prevention and education program, but very quickly realized that as important as education is, there was a lack of LGBT affirmative alcohol and drug abuse treatment. The bad news is that this absence still exists. Even after all these years, there is still a lot of hesitancy and resistance in mainstream alcohol and drug agencies, for example, to bringing LGBT issues out front. There is not as much overt homophobia as there used to be, but there is still bias, and so it is difficult to refer LGBT people to these programs if they felt that they were not free to be fully out. They may be tolerated as queer but not fully accepted. We used to quote Dr. Hellman's 1989 *Hospital and Community Psychiatry* study on attitudes and training in public treatment agencies.[2] Then, in 1998, the Manhattan Mental Health Federation's LGBT Community Advisory Committee repeated a somewhat similar version of it.[3] We interviewed 100 alcohol, drug, and mental health providers licensed by New York City. A person would call the program, acting as if they were a potential consumer inquiring about their services to LGBT individuals. Ninety-three had no LGBT specific services. For the 7 that did, the services consisted of an HIV support group. That was in 1998. So, 10 years after the Hellman study, it was still the case that public, mainstream alcohol, drug, and mental health agencies in New York City were not adequately providing LGBT sensitive clinical services.

JGLP: Were these programs providing services that were more specific to other cultural groups?

Dr. Warren: Yes, and that is what was appalling. Many of these programs were focused on being culturally competent in reflecting the diverse population of New York. But, when it came to LGBT issues, it did not seem to be the outright homophobia we encountered in the past. Instead, it was a lack of knowledge that it was important to acknowledge LGBT issues. So, it is less about hatred and more about negligence. There still seems to be an attitude of "it doesn't really matter, does it" and there is still a lack of understanding of how being LGBT is perceived in society, and what the barriers are for LGBT people in being out, accepting themselves, and being accepted. There is this myth now, because everybody watches television programs like *Will and Grace* or *Sex and the City*, that it is okay to be gay, and nobody has any problems with it anymore. They do not realize that there is still a lot of stigma, prejudice, and marginalization in our society that affects LGBT people, which coincides with race and class issues. So, we are still not there yet.

JGLP: The Center is not a clinic, but a community-based organization.

Dr. Warren: Yes, that is what is different about our programs. The services we provide came out of a community center, not a clinic or hospital, or a gay and lesbian program in a free-standing health center. The Center is an LGBT liberation organization that created services to help people who are active in that organization to be well, which is really a different orientation. We think our programs have been quite effective, and now we are trying to do some research to demonstrate that. People do not come to our programs so much as clients, more as participants. They end up being members of the Center, getting involved in the community and getting well in the community.

JGLP: So this model of intervention does not reinforce a "patient role?"

Dr. Warren: Right. It is about becoming empowered to be active in the community. It sounds hokey, but we have eighteen groups that are running at any given time out of our CenterCare program with 16-18 individuals in each 10 week cycle group. Why do so many people come to our groups? Because they are free or low-cost? Usually it is the other way around, where people more readily drop out of free groups. I think it is because it is the Center.

JGLP: What are the demographics of the population you serve?

Dr. Warren: There was an interesting myth among the different demographic groups here, where each felt that everybody else used the Center. So, many white gay men thought that mostly people of color used the Center, while the lesbians thought the Center was too dominated by gay men, and the gays thought that transgender and bisexual persons were underrepresented, and so on. The one group that everybody agreed did not take up much of the Center is the bisexual group, but, in fact, there are a number of bisexual groups that use the Center. As we grew, it became important to insure that everyone was more visible to everyone else, and to create programming to both reflect and accomplish a coming together of our diverse constituencies.

In fact, in our social service programs, our demographics basically are that more than 50% of participants are people of color, with about 25% African American, 20% Latino, and lesser percentages of Asian, Pacific Islanders, and Native Americans. In the Youth Program, 75% identify as young people of color, with 15-20% identifying as multi-racial.

JGLP: What about socioeconomic status?

Dr. Warren: This is a mixed bag, too. About 20% are living on some form of public assistance. It really runs the gamut. We have some very well off people who could easily afford private therapy, but they come to the Center because we have a reputation for providing quality services, and they want to be part of a group that is part of this community center.

JGLP: Do you think this sense of community can be found in the private sector?

Dr. Warren: Not really. We are like a settlement house. We used to nickname it the Gay Settlement House. I think that is a good analogy. Settlement houses were basically for immigrant groups who were displaced. Many of the LGBT people here came to New York because they could not be out in their local community. The Center became this oasis for them. They do not feel like they are coming to a clinic. They feel like they are coming to a community organization, and I think the fusion of this sense of community with the counseling services we offer is what makes this such a remarkable place. People come to feel that they are part of the Center family. We have such a diversity of people here with political and social differences. It is not so much a melting pot, but a place that serves as a catalyst for bringing people together to communicate and connect across differences.

JGLP: Who pays for your services?

Dr. Warren: Initially, it was all government and foundation grant funding, and of course, all of our donors. But it has gotten harder and harder to fund services through grants. Several years ago, we received a license as a prevention counseling program from the Office of Alcoholism and Substance Abuse Services as a first step, and now we are going to apply for a Chemical Dependency License so we can receive third party reimbursement. Our biggest service area is still substance abuse, and it is unfortunate that we do not have the capacity to subsidize our own services. Certainly, everybody else does, and yet they do not offer the type of culturally relevant services that we do.

We recently went to a sliding fee schedule for our groups. There was some fear at the beginning that people would not want to come, but then people actually said that it was about time we charged something. Now they feel that they are contributing something to the Center. People feel invested in this place. Some have expressed how it saved their life. They appreciate the staff and the services, and they want to give us something back.

The other thing that we did, and I will take some of the credit for this, was establish a training program for MSW, CASAC, and psychology interns. The value of offering quality training to students can never be underestimated. Many places with field placements just throw the student in with little supervision, and at the end of the placement, they feel that anything they learned was by accident. I am very oriented towards doing supervision and training, offering support and a meaningful experience. I also thought that LGBT students would really value an LGBT placement. We have 8-10 field placements a year, and I would say that about 50% of them end up working at the Center. So, providing this training has helped significantly in allowing us to offer the services we do.

JGLP: What about the relationships you established at city, state, and federal levels.

Dr. Warren: I think the thing that was most important was establishing a personal relationship with people at various levels of government. You can do good work, but if nobody knows about it, it is not going to get you far. Of course, you also have to be able to deliver based on what you ask for, or you will not be seen as credible. Richard Burns, our Executive Director, is very good at this. Personality is a part of it. Richard is articulate, passionate, and genuine, and seeks people out. I think that one of the reasons he hired me is that I have an affinity for creating those kind of relationships as well.

It is also about follow through. I am in an interesting position because I am not lesbian identified. One of the things that I noticed was that it was hard for LGBT individuals who were put in the position of having to go out and be the poster children. They were not just arguing for social justice. They were talking about their lives, and when people gave them grief about it, it could be very personally painful. I had this opportunity to be a little bit detached from it. Not detached in a way that I did not care, but I did not take it quite as personally, and so I could stay with it and not react to it.

This turned out to be quite beneficial when it came to our educational work with public health care agencies. I remember when I first started doing trainings with some very homophobic people in the health care business. We would sometimes be addressing a person that was quite angry and offensive. I have watched people do this in other lesbian and gay agencies, and, not unexpectedly, the trainer could become very edgy or intense. I was not in the same position, so I did not get defensive in the same way. I realized from these experiences that we would be working with very different people that had a range of attitudes. So, we decided to develop a team approach for this kind of work, where we would have a gay man, myself, a straight woman, a lesbian woman, a person of color, and so on. We would all come out in the training in terms of these identities, and role model working together, working across our differences. That really helped to set the right tone. People identify with their own experience, and we felt that if we could get them to identify with different backgrounds of people, and get them to identify with what it is like to be oppressed, regardless of why you are being oppressed, then maybe we could get them to join in the experience of fighting against marginalization across differences.

JGLP: Did the relationships you established with those in government translate into funding of your programs?

Dr. Warren: Absolutely. The bottom line is, when you have to write a competitive proposal, it can matter whom you know. When there are several good proposals out there, that can make the difference.

JGLP: Has the political climate affected the funding of LGBT programs?

Dr. Warren: Yes. First of all, the economic climate has. There are more and more people in the non-profit sector competing for less and less funding. Private giving has gone down, and states are now in an economic hole. There is now more competition for public dollars, particularly federal dollars, because state dollars have dried up to some extent.

Now, with the current federal administration under George Bush, faith-based initiatives are in the mix. All of a sudden, we are now competing with religious organizations that were not allowed to apply before. People say, "oh, it's such a small percentage," but I review proposals for the federal government, and there are actually a lot of religious organizations that are now applying that were not competing with us in the past. There is a willingness to want to give faith based organizations some of those dollars. The other thing that people say is, "oh, it's a competitive proposal," so the highest score wins. But, this is not so. There is a geographic consideration, a demographic consideration, and now a faith-related consideration. If there are five grants and ten good proposals, one might go the east coast, one to the west coast, and now one to a faith-based organization, so the competition is tougher.

JGLP: What would you say has been the most significant barrier in developing and realizing your program?

Dr. Warren: Two things. One is the persistent notion among well meaning people that the best thing they can do for LGBT people is to say that we are all equal and it does not matter. Here, we are dealing with the mistaken notion that the way to LGBT equality is to make us all the same.

The other barrier that acts in tandem with that has to do with a vociferous and calculated campaign from the radical right in this country to undermine LGBT issues. In many cases, I do not think they care one way or another about LGBT issues, but they use it as a way to consolidate their political power and have influence. Because of this, many politicians and leaders that might have a favorable opinion about LGBT issues will not take a stand regarding LGBT affirmative policies. The Clinton administration gave more access to LGBT people at the highest levels of government than ever in the history of this country. But at the same time, they tried to offset their issues with the radical right by taking an antigay marriage stand, and the "Don't Ask, Don't Tell" stand.

These have been two of the hardest issues to overcome, and what happens in terms of funding, is that it just becomes easier to fund, say, a woman's cancer program. But, of course, not a lesbian cancer program since that is part of that "lesbian agenda."

JGLP: Considering these realities, what strategies have worked well?

Dr. Warren: Cultivating personal relationships, not "burning bridges." Finding some way for the other person to join or connect with you, no matter how different their views. It is hard sometimes. It is important for certain people in the community to take a stand. Richard Burns taught me how in trying to fund and finance to keep the movement going, you sometimes feel that you have to do things that might compromise your integrity. I do not pander to others, but sometimes you have to be less than out front with certain folks, because you want to engage them, and not alienate them. It is sometimes a real challenge to find the right balance where you can open a door without compromising your integrity.

JGLP: How far would you say we have come in terms of the provision of public mental health services to the LGBT community?

Dr. Warren: Tremendously far, and yet "so near, yet so far." There really has been a positive cultural shift in this country in the last ten years regarding the perception of LGBT people. By the same token, it still astounds me as to the degree to which there is still stigma out there, and an unwillingness in many places to accept LGBT identity as a normal and integral part of the societal whole.

As an example, I am currently working on the issue of tobacco cessation. New York State is about to implement the Adult Tobacco Surveillance Survey (ATS). It is a standardized instrument that utilizes a structured interview, administered via random telephone dialing. It is an effort to determine the prevalence of tobacco use in the population, why people smoke, if they are accessing preventive or cessation programs, and how successful they are. Tobacco money is currently funding so many other things, and this is a way of demonstrating that there is a need for some of the tobacco settlement money to go into this program area, especially since tobacco related illness is the leading cause of preventable death in this country. It far outweighs cancer, heart disease, and AIDS. It is the leading cause of preventable death in the LGBT community. Furthermore, those with psychiatric disorders are twice as likely to smoke as others, according to research by Karen Lasser published in the *Journal of the American Medical Association* in November, 2000.[4] New York has actually been fairly progressive in the tobacco field, and there are a number of LGBT people at the forefront in this effort.

The Center has one of the high profile LGBT tobacco cessation programs. The NYS Department of Health's Tobacco Control program is about ready to run this instrument in New York, so I send the DOH an e-mail asking if they have included a question on sexual orientation or gender identity on the ATS. The response was that they were "considering" the addition of such a question.

You ask how much things have changed, and here we are in a country where we still do not collect data on sexual orientation or gender identity when we ask about health care issues. So, when it comes time to allocate funding to particular health care initiatives, the government uses the demographics in these general surveys. And, because of this type of omission, we hear officials tell us that there is no evidence about that. We have pointed out to them that they do not ask about sexual identity, so it is a real Catch-22.

So, the survey people send me a sample of the question they are considering. The question was, "Are you homosexual?" And I thought, "Oh, my. They are not going to get a lot of useful information from that." Well, we were able to offer input into a better way to get at these demographics. And, at this point, I think this is going to be revolutionary for a large survey of this kind. They are going to ask three questions: (1) how do you best describe your identity: as gay, lesbian, bisexual, heterosexual, or "other;" (2) if you identify as male, female, or "other;" and, (3) if you also identify as transgender. I am thrilled and tell them they are now on the cutting edge for a national survey. But, then I get a response just before their pilot test about consent forms, inquiring whether they should inform people up front that they are going to ask about their sexual orientation, because won't that turn them off, and they will not consent to take the survey?

The point is that even survey researchers who are progressive, are still worried that people will be offended by the sexual orientation questions. I responded saying, "Bite the bullet." If you act like it is normal, they will respond as if it is normal to ask. If you act like there is something wrong with asking the questions, and your phrasing reflects that, they will respond in kind. Just be matter-of-fact in your consent form and say, "We are going to ask you questions about your gender, gender identity, sexual orientation, race, and ethnicity. If you act in a matter-of-fact way, people will end up thinking that way." I think that is the kind of struggle which causes us so much frustration.

JGLP: In your view, what other clinical, organizational, or political challenges lie ahead?

Dr. Warren: Back in the 50s and 60s, the civil rights movement gained momentum, and then a lot of white people joined in. I am not sure that the LGBT movement has had the same support from straight people. I am not sure why. There have been a number of times, say for example, when Matthew Shepard was murdered, that I thought, "Now it is going to happen. Now there will be a straight civil rights organization for queer justice." There were a lot of straight young people who took up the gauntlet at that time, but then it just faded. Maybe it was because there seemed to be so many affluent gay people that had become visible, and it did not appear that the LGBT community was oppressed anymore. I do not know how to explain this, but it is disappointing. I know that I have been able to do some significant work by role modeling as a heterosexual woman who is also a "queer" social justice activist.

JGLP: Do you have any thoughts about establishing standards for LGBT mental health training and clinical services?

Dr. Warren: As I think you know, many of us have been working on that for years. Yet, at present, I think we continue to struggle politically to establish why there is a wider need for this. We are still struggling with the notion that all you have to do is provide good services that everyone has access to, and not to "ghetto-ize" services by establishing special LGBT programs. Of course, on the political right, establishing such standards is viewed as part of the "homosexual conspiracy." That has been part of the problem in getting mainstream programs to acknowledge that we need sensitivity trainings and LGBT-oriented approaches.

We had been working at the federal level on developing a training program that was funded during the Clinton administration, and I am not sure that it will be released during the Bush administration. But, it was definitely paid for, and

I was one of the people who worked on it. This was a project to develop a national curriculum on LGBT sensitivity for alcohol, drug, and mental health treatment programs. We have been trying for years to have cultural competency regulations that programs must comply with, and that are reviewed in audits for city and state licensure renewal. These regulations would mandate training in sexual orientation and gender identity. But quite frankly, I think it needs to be legislated like affirmative action.

JGLP: So, the public sector, and specifically government, needs to be in the vanguard in this area?

Dr. Warren: Yes, and in certain ways, some people have been part of this. People in both public agencies and political leaders have pushed for this. There are some very good people behind the scenes who are not very well known that are involved in this effort. A good example is Don Burger. He is a straight-identified man who is just about to retire. He has worked in the Professional Training Division of the New York State Office of Alcoholism and Substance Abuse Services for 20 years. He was a staunch ally regarding the inclusion of LGBT training, and New York State produced the first-ever state manual to train clinicians and administrators on LGBT issues in substance abuse.

The federal government subsequently modeled a providers guide based on this manual. This happened years ago because Don Burger championed it from the inside, and he was in a position to allocate some funding. It got some resistance, but he had been there for 20 years. He had some autonomy, and he went ahead and did it. He convened the work group, brought us up to Albany, paid for us to develop the training, put it in the New York State training curriculum, advertised it, had us train the trainers, and it became part of the training curriculum. We brought it to the Clinton administration, where the Substance Abuse and Mental Health Services Administration (SAMHSA) "oohed and aahed" over it. New York State was quite proud of this, but Don Burger was really why it happened. He just went ahead and did it.

JGLP: So, sometimes it just takes one individual's initiative?

Dr. Warren: Yes, but the thing about Don Burger is that he had lots of LGBT colleagues whom he trusted to help develop something meaningful that would stand up to scrutiny. If it had been a weak curriculum, it would have gotten enough opposition to crumble. It held up because he knew the right people to ask to help him develop it. So, it always works both ways. He was on the inside, but he knew others that could help him do something credible.

JGLP: Any final thoughts about the lessons you have learned over the years in developing and administering LGBT programs in the public sector?

Dr. Warren: Again, I would emphasize the relationship building. You can never tell who will go on to become a friend and ally, so you have to stay open to the possibility that people who initially do not seem likely, may end up "getting it." Also, I would keep in mind that there are many levels involved, and you do not want to get stuck on any one level. You have to think not only about the front line of service delivery, but also about policy at the municipal, state, and federal levels. We have had many successes at coalition building and collaboration. Over the years, I have learned that it is much harder to collaborate than to do it yourself. There are benefits to both, but in the long run, the collaborations take longer and are harder to pull off, but they always end up being more beneficial. Patience, and a willingness to quietly listen across differences can result in the least likely person becoming your staunchest ally.

NOTES

1. New York State Office of Alcoholism and Substance Abuse Services (1996), *Working with Lesbian, Gay, Bisexual and Transgender Persons in Alcoholism and Substance Abuse Services.* Albany: New York State Office of Alcoholism and Substance Abuse Services.

2. Hellman, R., Stanton, M., Lee, J., Tytun, A. & Vachon, R. (1989), Treatment of homosexual alcoholics in government-funded agencies: Provider training and attitudes. *Hospital & Community Psychiatry,* 40:1163-1168.

3. Lesbian, Gay, Bisexual, Transgender Hygiene Issues Committee (1998), New York City Federation for Mental Health, Mental Retardation, and Alcoholism Services. Unpublished survey.

4. Lasser, K., Boyd, J.W., Woolhandler, S., Himmelstein, D.U., McCormick, D. & Bor, D.H. (2000), Smoking and mental illness: A population-based prevalence study. *JAMA,* 284:2606-2610.

Index

BOOK ORDER FORM!

Order a copy of this book with this form or online at:
http://www.haworthpress.com/store/product.asp?sku=5363

Handbook of LGBT Issues
in Community Mental Health

___ in softbound at $24.95 (ISBN: 0-7890-2310-5)
___ in hardbound at $49.95 (ISBN: 0-7890-2309-1)

COST OF BOOKS _____	❑ **BILL ME LATER:**
	Bill-me option is good on US/Canada/ Mexico orders only; not good to jobbers, wholesalers, or subscription agencies.
POSTAGE & HANDLING _____	
US: $4.00 for first book & $1.50 for each additional book.	❑ **Signature** _____
Outside US: $5.00 for first book & $2.00 for each additional book.	❑ **Payment Enclosed: $** _____
SUBTOTAL _____	❑ **PLEASE CHARGE TO MY CREDIT CARD:**
In Canada: add 7% GST. _____	❑ Visa ❑ MasterCard ❑ AmEx ❑ Discover
STATE TAX _____	❑ Diner's Club ❑ Eurocard ❑ JCB
CA, IL, IN, MN, NJ, NY, OH & SD residents please add appropriate local sales tax.	**Account #** _____
FINAL TOTAL _____	**Exp Date** _____
If paying in Canadian funds, convert using the current exchange rate, UNESCO coupons welcome.	**Signature** _____
	(Prices in US dollars and subject to change without notice.)

PLEASE PRINT ALL INFORMATION OR ATTACH YOUR BUSINESS CARD

Name

Address

City   State/Province   Zip/Postal Code

Country

Tel   Fax

E-Mail

May we use your e-mail address for confirmations and other types of information? ❑ Yes ❑ No We appreciate receiving your e-mail address. Haworth would like to e-mail special discount offers to you, as a preferred customer. **We will never share, rent, or exchange your e-mail address.** We regard such actions as an invasion of your privacy.

Order From Your **Local Bookstore** or Directly From
The Haworth Press, Inc. 10 Alice Street, Binghamton, New York 13904-1580 • USA
Call Our toll-free number (1-800-429-6784) / Outside US/Canada: (607) 722-5857
Fax: 1-800-895-0582 / Outside US/Canada: (607) 771-0012
E-mail your order to us: orders@haworthpress.com

For orders outside US and Canada, you may wish to order through your local
sales representative, distributor, or bookseller.
For information, see http://haworthpress.com/distributors

(Discounts are available for individual orders in US and Canada only, not booksellers/distributors.)

Please photocopy this form for your personal use.
www.HaworthPress.com

BOF04